Women

on

Childbirth

Women on Childbirth: tips and experiences from women who have done it.

Women on Childbirth is an essential book for any woman expecting a baby. From caesarean sections to natural births, no matter how you choose to give birth, one of these women have done it before. Catherine Balavage had a traumatic birth with her first child, which spurred her on to talk to other women about their experiences and find out more about childbirth. She then went on to have a successful VBAC (vaginal birth after caesarean) with her second child. Women on Childbirth aims to empower woman with stories of childbirth, but also provide tips and information. It is essential reading for any woman who is going to give birth.

Edited By: Catherine Balavage

First published in 2017

Copyright © Catherine Balavage 2017

Disclaimer

The information provided in this book is designed to provide information on the subjects discussed. This book is not meant to be used, nor should it be used, as medical advice.

This book is not an endorsement of any particular birthing technique. The content of each chapter is the sole expression and opinion of its author, and not necessarily that of the editor or publisher. You should consult a licenced physician to discuss your different options prior to your birth.

By reading this book, you accept that the publisher, authors and editor are not responsible for your birth and are not liable for any damages or negative consequences that may result from any treatment, action, or preparation.

References are provided for informational purposes only and do not constitute endorsement of any websites or other sources. Readers should be aware that the websites listed in this book may change. In addition, the authors, editor and publisher do not represent or warrant that the information accessible via this book is accurate, complete or current.

Use of this book implies your acceptance of this disclaimer.

For Luke and Sophia

Contents List

Introduction...4

Rachel Thamm 7

Alexandra Bannard 10

Glo Butane...22

My Birth Experiences by Paola Bagnall......................................23

N D Hardwick

"Paracetamol My Dear?"..26

My Birth Story

by Rachel Braun: Audrey...28

The Best Father's Day Present

by Motherhudds

34 weeks..32

My Birth Stories by Louise George 40

By Becky O'Haire, Cuddle Fairy Blog..46

Knife to Skin. My Birth Story by Catherine Balavage 52

Milli Hill of The Positive Birth Movement....................................58

Top Ten tips on How to Use Self-Hypnosis for Birth Hypnobirthing

By Paola Bagnall..60

Why a Caesarean Can be a Positive Birth Experience by Catherine Balavage 64

   The Stages of Labour 64

Some Awesome Tips Unrelated to the Topic of the Book..................66

   Different Types of Births..66

   Pain Relief Options 67

   Recovering After Birth..67

   What You Will Need 68

Introduction

As I write this introduction, my daughter Sophia is asleep in her Moses basket. The run up to her birth was an anxious time. The memories of the traumatic birth of her brother were still with me, always sitting at the edge of my mind. I knew I would be unlucky to go through the same thing again, and that no two births are the same, but the unpredictably of childbirth played on my mind. I worried about having another C-section, but I was also worried that I was being selfish trying to have a VBAC (vaginal birth after caesarean). Friends told me I was crazy, *'why go through childbirth again?'* they asked. I wondered the same thing myself. But I decided to keep the faith. I interviewed other women for their stories, talked to midwives and read every book on childbirth I could find. I decided to be as prepared as possible while knowing that a birth plan is merely a wish. There is no planning. But there is preparation. And there are things you can do to improve your chances of a good birth and a quicker recovery.

When I got scared or anxious about the birth, I reminded myself that all pain is temporary and that my son was worth every second of the pain I went through with his birth. It is quite common for women who go through a traumatic birth to become obsessed with birth. To read up on it as much as possible. I was no exception.

Childbirth. It is one word which always provokes a reaction. We all know childbirth is a wee bit hurty. People say something was '*like childbirth*', when they are trying to convey how painful something was. They also use it when they talk about putting themselves through that pain again. Except the last part is not really true. You do not forget, you just know that every moment of it was worth it. When I was growing up, my mother always described childbirth as, *'so painful you feel like you are dying, then it is so painful you want to die, and then it is over.'* It is a miracle the woman has any grandchildren at all.

So, when we think about childbirth we think about pain, but I wanted to write this book because childbirth is not about pain and it does not need to be terrifying. It is okay to be nervous and I am not going to lie and say it does not hurt, but everything in life that is worth having tends to bring some suffering, big or small.

Childbirth used to be shrouded in mystery and women did not have full access to their rights. It used to be something that no one talked about. Now there are television programmes such as '*One Born Every Minute'* and '*Call the Midwife'*. Childbirth is part of the national conversation.

Mummy bloggers have opened up a new era of honest parenting. There are numerous books on childbirth and internet forums like '*Mumsnet*' and '*Netmums*' to enable women to seek support, no matter what time of the day, no matter what the issue. It is fair to say that women are not alone; there is an entire community out there. However, sometimes it can feel like we have the opposite problem: that we are now drowning in information. I wanted to put this book together because my own childbirth experience was traumatic. I needed to heal and the research helped, as did talking to other women. Although my own experience was awful, in a way I was lucky. I still managed to bond with my child.

Many women suffer with post-natal depression and many women find it hard to bond. Others struggle to breastfeed. There are no right or wrong answers. There are just women all struggling to get through the day, full of hormones and feeling like they've been hit by a truck - both physically and emotionally. But we are not alone. Not anymore. We have each other. Since becoming a mother, the best thing I have discovered is just how supportive women are to each other. The level of support has been unbelievable. We tell each other stories and we can relate to them. We give advice and support. I have been almost reduced to tears by just how kind people are: doctors, midwives (mostly!), nurses, health visitors; all of these people went beyond any sense of normal duty and saved my life many times over.

The real difference in my life was when I started going to baby and toddler groups. I know, I know, when am I going to get to the childbirth bit, but you need to know this. Go to toddler groups. Go to baby groups. Go to soft play. You will not want to leave the house some days. Most days in fact, but it will save your life because the people there will be amazing and supportive, including the mums, dads, grandparents and staff. Talk to as many other mothers as possible. Invite them for coffee or lunch. Join '*Mush*' or other apps that bring mothers together. But this is all after the topic we are to talk about. Let's go back to the task in hand. I cannot promise there will be no diversions because I have some advice to give. I am going to bring you excellent birth stories from wonderful writers, but I am also going to give you advice on childbirth. There is also some advice on how to cope as a new parent. So, congratulations on the start of a new, amazing journey. Nothing is as amazing as the moment they place your baby on your chest and nothing is more glorious, scary, wonderful, brilliant, chaotic, awful, exhausting, relentless or miraculous as becoming a mother. It is the best thing ever. But first you have to push that baby out. So here we go.

Out of all of the books I have written this has been the hardest. Not just because there were so many contributors, but because my own birth story was not a happy one. The outcome was happy, but the birth itself was a catalogue of errors. I had a traumatic birth. I requested a birth review with the hospital and was left even more infuriated. They would not take responsibility at all. The first thing they said was, '*you had a lot of drugs, didn't you?*' Well, given I was in labour for five days, yeah, of course I bloody did. But I digress, that is for later.

I am not a doctor or a midwife. Nothing I give is medical advice and should not be taken as such. I am a writer and I do what writers do: research, find the facts, and talk to experts. I then take this research and put it all together. That is what I have done here. I have found some amazing women to share their birth stories, while also including the information you need for your birth. I hope this book helps you. I hope it makes you feel less nervous and more prepared. It can be the loss of control that makes childbirth so scary. My second birth was a drug free VBAC (vaginal birth after previous caesarean). As painful as it was at the time, it was a healing process. I now know my body can give birth and that what happened before was not my fault. I am glad I decided on that path and it worked out for me, but I think even more importantly, it is critical that if it had not happened that I did not beat myself up about it. The only person who can make the right choices on how you give birth is you. '*Good for her, not for me,*' should be everyone's mantra. I hope this book entertains and educates. I also hope it helps you make the right choices for you. So, read on and feel more prepared.

The Amazing Contributors Who I Love and Thank

Rachel Thamm

Alexandra Bannard

Glo Butane

Paola Bagnall - Author and Hypnobirthing Teacher.

N D Hardwick - *www.mumthemagician.com*

Rachel Braun - www.mywildjourney.com.

MotherHudds - MotherHudds runs a social media site for mums in Huddersfield. https://twitter.com/motherhudds

Louise George - http://littleheartsbiglove.co.uk.

Becky O'Haire - Cuddle Fairy Blog, www.cuddlefairy.com

Reneé Davis Wife - mama, author, blogger http://mummytries.com

Catherine Balavage - Author and Editor of http://www.frostmagazine.com

Milli Hill of The Positive Birth Movement - http://www.positivebirthmovement.org

Rachel Thamm

I can't believe how time as flown, given that nearly twenty-two years ago, at the age of twenty-one, I had my first child, inherited a couple from my husband Mark and then had two more in my thirties. My '*baby*' turns eleven this year but I swear he was just born the other day!

This is his story….

Ashton Philip John Thamm

In 1993 I had Keelin, who arrived in about three hours and weighed a healthy 7.7lb (3.5kg). This was followed by Brooke in 2001, who weighed just under 10lb (4kg) and arrived in only one hour and fifty minutes. Both pregnancies were REVOLTING with constant sickness throughout and after Brooke, we decided not to have any more. But in October 2003 there happened one night in Las Vegas, a wedding chapel and a bottle of Tequila…. but alas, that is another story.

So, in December 2003 the morning sickness started, then the all-day sickness. It is actually hard to describe how miserable you feel carrying the nausea around with you, unable to sit, relax and enjoy things due to the constant nagging sickness. As I had experienced with Brooke and Keelin, I ended up back in hospital several times with dehydration whilst carrying Ashton. I didn't know that Ashton was a boy at this stage and I must admit that given we had all the *girly* things and I had exactly the same pregnancy symptoms, I was really convinced it was another girl. Oh boy, was I in for a surprise! Eventually the doctors put me on Ondansetron to try and reduce the vomiting and nausea. I tried not to take them as much as possible, as I was really worried about having medication whilst pregnant, however, I also knew that the strain of being constantly ill was damaging my body.

When I was about seven months pregnant I was driving to my obstetrics appointment when I heard on the radio that the Government were going to pay a '*baby bonus*'. I'm one who believes that things happen for a reason so, when a brochure flew off the shelf and hit me while I was booking into my appointment, I took notice. It was a brochure for a cryogenics company for cord blood storage. Not a big deal except I saw that the price was EXACTLY, to the dollar, the same amount as the baby bonus I had just heard on the radio. So, after a discussion with my doctor, we decided to collect the cord blood. My doctor had not done this before and was sent into a mild panic at the thought of making a mistake, so I was regaled with stories of how he was practicing with his wife and a glove, even though I REALLY didn't want to know. It also meant that I had to reduce any drugs taken during birth (I am a BIG fan of the epidural) – but I decided that given how quick Brooke's birth had taken, I thought I would be able to manage without pain relief for this birth. I am looking back wondering if I wasn't slightly delusional from the illness….

My doctor advised that the baby was about the same size as Brooke and would be around ten pounds, however, from about thirty-four weeks I found it hard to catch my breath. I wondered if it was the Ondansetron (anti-nausea) medication. I was constantly worried that my illness and the medication would harm my baby so at thirty-six weeks I stopped all medication. At forty weeks and two days the doctors finally decided to induce me. In hindsight I should have been induced several weeks earlier.

So, into the hospital we went, expecting that we would have our new little girl in a couple of hours. After checking in, getting our room and meeting the staff, the induction gel (Prostaglandan) was inserted and rubbed on the bottom of my cervix by the midwife. This started contractions within about fifteen minutes and after about thirty minutes my cervix was starting to dilate nicely and my waters broke within the hour. I was managing the pain like a trooper. (Ok, I was bloody regretting my decision to go drug free after about ten minutes.)

After ten hours my labour was still going and I was completely exhausted. I felt like the baby was stuck and no matter how hard I pushed, I couldn't seem to get any further along. My doctor came back around 10.00pm and I had been now been in labour for about twelve hours. My husband tells me that he learnt some new and very creative swear words from me during this time. The doctor had a look and told us that the baby was presenting with one arm extended (think Superman) and was pushing himself back. The doctor and my husband then thought it would be funny to commentate on the action, '*here he comes, nahhhhh there he goes*'; '*here he comes, nahhhh there goes*'. After about fifteen minutes of this I very politely told them that they were Asshats and I would get off the bed and bang their heads together if they said another word. Ever.

I understand now they were both just trying to get me fired up a bit so that we could get this baby out. It worked and my doctor spent the next hour or so slowly turning the baby so that it could be delivered safely. This consisted of many '*push*', '*don't push*' instructions and about a billion swear words from me. My poor husband also got a verbal tirade about the size of his big, fat head on several occasions. The nursing staff told me afterwards that it was the best job they had ever seen and that if I hadn't had such a good doctor I would have been ripped to shreds – not a pleasant thing to consider but made me feel glad I went with my gut in selecting this one.

Finally, after nearly fifteen hours, at 12.40am, the baby was born and my doctor began harvesting the cord blood for collection. On being told it was a boy I can still remember thinking, '*that would be bloody right*'. I caught the doctor and my husband looking at each other and became concerned that there was something wrong. It turns out they were both shocked as Ashton was 56cm long, his head was nearly 40cm and he weighed in at 5.36kg which is just under 12lb. WOW.

It was no wonder I was struggling to get my breath for the last few months, there just wasn't any room left for my poor lungs.

The doctor was worried that he hadn't collected the cord blood correctly, or hadn't collected enough, but it turns out that he collected twice the amount we were able to store so we were able to donate some for others to use.

I still remember being asked why we were '*back in the hospital*' and if Ashton was sick and having to convince the other new mothers that he was a new-born – he was a giant!

My Tips for Birth and Labour are Quite Simple – it's all about you:

- You need to be comfortable and trust your doctor or midwife. Pre-agree levels of 'intervention' i.e. are your comfortable with forceps or ventouse and under what circumstances would they be used. I prefer the doctor to turn the baby and get it out naturally if possible, but this isn't always the case – ask questions and be happy with the answers or find another specialist.

- You need to have support during the birth, (don't be afraid to kick your husband to the curb and get a friend or parent in or have a tag team as it is exhausting for them as well). If you wouldn't go to the toilet in front of the person, then do yourself a favour and choose someone else, as there is no room for embarrassment during a birth.

- Be comfortable, wear what you want and create a nice environment, play music if you want, television, a massage – it is your time so be demanding!

- Have pain relief! Don't let others tell you what to do and what not to do. It doesn't hurt the baby and you will be bloody glad you chose it.

- It is going to be messy. Don't worry about it. It is nothing they haven't seen hundreds of times.

- Rub nipple cream on before the baby is born to prevent the chafing once they start to feed. Breast feeding is not EASY – I have no idea why but it isn't. Some babies are really hard to get on the nipple, keep trying, keep trying, it will happen.

- Drink lots of water.

- Wrap or don't wrap, dummy or no dummy – you're the parent, you chose.

- Do your pelvic floor exercises, and yes, they are crappy but in ten years when you cough and don't wet your pants you will be grateful.

- Don't be supermum, get others to help as sleep is a precious diamond – if you don't need to be doing it then don't, delegate it.

- Make noise at home, get your baby used to sleeping with noise. When they get older they will be able to sleep anywhere – much nicer than having to race home every time they need a nap.

- Enjoy your baby – they are bloody hard work but take time out just to look at them and marvel at what you created. They are really cute when they are sleeping!

Rachel Thamm Biography

I am currently a National Human Resources Manager in the energy industry, a long journey from my beginnings in 1990 as a Police Officer on the beat in South Australia. Leaving the Police force in 2001 I started my own workplace investigation consultancy firm and was also lecturing Emergency Management at University. In 2010 I decided I needed a change, however, it wasn't until 2012 when I was offered my current role, that I actually made the jump. Whilst my salary took a sharp nose dive, the increase in my happiness was well worth the pain – I love my job and feel incredibly lucky to have found such a great place to work.

Alexandra Bannard

My Kuwait Birthing Story

Before I had my kids, I thought giving birth was the most natural thing in the world. Of course, the reality is something different. Even in Western nations, maternal mortality was the biggest killer of healthy women as late as the 1950's and in many less fortunate countries, it is still responsible for more deaths in otherwise healthy women than anything else.

But this is not what my story is about. As soon as I became a mum I realized everyone had a unique birthing story and I became fascinated with and intrigued by them. This is my own account of what it is like giving birth in a foreign country, warts and all.

We were living in Kuwait when I discovered I was pregnant. We were engaged but not yet married and so the news of my pregnancy was greeted with an f-bomb instead of joy and elation. It was not the ideal response but marginally better than, '*Is it mine?*'

Kuwait is a relatively strict Muslim state. Technically, we should not have even been living together, let alone getting up the duff together, so the first thing to do was to go straight to the British Embassy and register our banns. A month later in a ministry office with a pink fluffy heart atop the pen, a token gesture of romance, I asked Mr P for his permission to marry him (such is the Islamic ritual), much to the merriment of our male friends who were there to witness this not so romantic of ceremonies. Straight after, we hotfooted it to the hospital to meet a doctor where we saw our baby, who was sucking his thumb, and discovered he was fourteen weeks old already, the first trimester had passed me by almost unnoticed.

When we told friends the happy news, some of whom were midwives in another hospital in Kuwait, they went grey when we told them who our Obs & Gynae doctor was. *"We sacked her from our hospital, please go anywhere, any hospital, it doesn't have to be ours but don't use THAT woman, she is a liability, please,'* they implored. Again, not quite the response I had imagined but I am forever grateful for their candour.

The next day we went straight to The Royal Hyatt to meet with Dr Marcus and have a look around. We were smitten immediately. Hospitals in the Middle East are often more like hotels, the private rooms ranging from something typically upmarket resort 5-star, to 7-star glitz and glamour. Nothing less for the Middle Eastern princesses, you know.

Dr Marcus was reassuring and professional, Maltese originally but he had practiced for a long time in the UK so he got our sense of humour and I knew we had made the right decision.

As my due date neared, my amniotic fluid levels began to decline. Every week I went in to be checked; if they fell too low, I was to be induced. Thankfully, we threw a Christmas party and I spent a week organizing 8,000-odd iTunes tracks into playlists for the party and my fluid levels stabilized - because I was actually not running around like a mentalist for once.

By Christmas Eve, five days before the due date, Elbo, as he was known in-vetro, was being monitored.

'Oh,' says Dr Marcus, 'You're in labour.'

'Really? I thought they were Branston Pickles?' I replied using our colloquialism for Brakston Hicks contractions.

'Nope, the real deal,' said the man who should know.

'Right....what does that mean?' I asked. I mean, really...where had I been during those prenatal sessions?

'Not that much until you are 7-8cms dilated to be honest,' replied the doc, 'but do me a favour, I could really do with a day off tomorrow so take it slow.'

That evening we were having Christmas drinks, (illegal, Kuwait is a dry state, you see) where everyone tried to guess Elbo's ETA, whilst I winced at the occasional contraction. But since my waters hadn't broken, nothing seemed imminent.

Of course, I spent the night wide awake with contractions every ten minutes but nothing I couldn't handle and I was feeling optimistic that my *skipping-through-delivery-in-my-white-linen-dress-daisies-in-my-hands, au naturelle* birthing plan would go swimmingly. On Christmas Day, with the hubster at work in the morning (they don't celebrate Christmas in Kuwait), I even wandered slowly over to the shopping mall to pick up some last-minute Christmas gifts.

After Mr P finished work we were lunching with friends and I was not allowed in the car unless my hospital bag was packed and coming with us. The afternoon went much to plan;

a lovely Christmas lunch which I could eat, so no dramas, the occasional wince of ouch-ness and a glass or two of vino (well the midwife at the antenatal classes had said when labour starts, have a glass of wine and she should know).

Late afternoon my friend's husband started timing my contractions and eventually announced, '*wow they are five minutes apart, now.*' I looked horrified and my friend, who is a mother of two and therefore in my eyes an expert, suggested I call the hospital, who advised me to come in. I finished the wine and off hubster and I set. With hindsight maybe they just wanted to get rid of us?

In the waiting room, I looked rather smugly at my husband as we could hear screams of pain from behind closed doors, I must have had an expression of, '*I've SO got this',* written all over my face.

My contractions had slowed down by this time to 7-8 minutes apart, probably as the old fight or flight hormones kicked in, but I was told they were going to admit me for the night. Then our three Irish midwife friends arrived and announced they had made a pact to get us through the birth. Wow, I was SO touched and a little relieved that I hadn't known in advance; oh, the stage fright at the thought of my mates seeing my bits.

They then produced a large bottle of Volvic filled with vodka and proceeded, in true Irish style, to celebrate Christmas with my husband. Did I mention that it was like a rather awful episode of Father Ted, except instead of three drunk vicars, we had three drunk midwives?

After a while, I got restless and had forgotten all my best laid plans: no child's pose, zero walking around between contractions and staying on all fours during contractions absolutely did not happen, so I asked the girls if anything was going to happen tonight.

'*Oh, to be sure nothin' will be happening tonight Alex, you'll be grand,*' and other such gorgeous Irish platitudes. I am a sucker for an accent, especially an Irish accent.

'Can I go home then please?' I ventured.

Mr P looked slightly horrified that his impromptu piss-up with his mates might go south and the girls looked bemused, but a quick call to the lovely Dr Marcus and yep, I was good to go.

Of course, as soon as I got home and Mr P drifted off to sleep, god forbid he should lose a minute's sleep during this debacle, the contractions cranked up to four minutes apart. I was on and off that birthing ball like a woman possessed. I had the tens machine on and off to a barrage of foul-mouthed insults, useless contraption it was.

By 2.00am, *au naturelle* birthing my arse, I wanted drugs, all of them, so I called my midwife friends who were, to use the technical Irish term, lamped - absolutely wasted.

'Go back in,' they advised, no they slurred, 'they will give you whatever you want.'

'No, I can't do that, I discharged myself,' I insisted, 'I'll go in the morning but I just need to know it won't be too late by then.'

'No, you'll be grand, to be sure.'

When Mr P awoke I was bouncing on that bloody ball ready to throw that ruddy tens machine out of the window. 'Ready to try again?' he chirped all refreshed from a good night's sleep.

'Yes...' I sighed.

Of course, when we arrived at the hospital, the contractions slowed down again to seven minutes and the doctor on duty merrily announced that I was no further dilated and suggested I to go for a nice long walk. What? Are you mental? After twelve hours of four-minute contractions and I am no further forward? I am not going for a sodding walk, I can barely stand. Obviously, this was all in my head, I was still at that point remaining quite British and polite. She gave me a sweep instead. Oh, the indignity, the pain. Let's just say it made my eyes water, my blood boil and sent my expletive ridden mind into overdrive.

Dr Marcus arrived and asked how our Christmas was and we got derailed for a moment with pleasantries. Then we got back down to business. He announced that he would try a gel, '*which will either speed things along nicely...or not.*' If not, then apparently, we just had to wait it out until Elbo was ready to greet us.

I wasn't that optimistic to be honest, given the way things had progressed so far and that my waters were still in situ. Then the gel kicked in. I now know I was being induced, I am glad I didn't know then because I had heard horror stories about this. Actually, I think the term is augmentation once you are in labour. Anyway, whatever the term, that was me and it was working.

I have honestly never known anything like it. It was like going into labour on the back of a rocket ship. The contractions were so intense and were literally back-to-back, there was no respite. If I'm really honest I thought I was probably dying. Thankfully the girls, who were back and had been inhaling a cooked breakfast with real bacon in the corner with Mr P, knew what to expect and had the anaesthesiologist pop in as soon as she was free. It was probably only half an hour of endless excruciating pain but long enough. She inserted the epidural and almost immediately, all was good in my world again.

With hindsight, I guess the tone of the room changed but at the time I only knew something was potentially happening when I asked for a coffee and was told, no I wouldn't be needing a coffee. Oh, good I thought, finally I'm not dying and we are actually making some progress here.

At some point someone broke my waters and then Dr Marcus arrived looking a little serious. He explained that the baby was in distress, I was losing a lot of blood and showed me something that looked suspiciously like my womb from somewhere let's just say south of the border, (TMI doc, TMI) and that we needed to go in for an emergency C-section immediately. He added, 'I know it's not what you wanted but we have to do it now.'

Just then the girls swung in in their operating finest. I mean it was impressive and not unlike an episode of ER, but without the revolving cameras and George of the Cloonster, sadly.

Mr P, who was probably too busy finishing off his breakfast, missed it all and someone had to explain to him what was going on as he was whisked off for his swabs. I looked imploringly at Noreen and said, 'He will be okay, won't he?' meaning of course Elbo, not Mr P.

'We have to get him out, I can't make any promises, we have to get him out,' was her not very reassuring reply. She wasn't unfortunately talking about Mr P either.

As they wheeled me to theatre I looked at up at Mr P, the fear in his eyes matching the fear I knew was swimming in mine.

Thereafter, it was all incredibly quick. I was asked if I could feel the ice. 'What ice?' I replied and looked down to see ice on my arms. I couldn't feel anything.

In truth, I could hardly breathe. It felt like someone was sitting on my chest but I knew we couldn't waste any time on me, we had to get Elbo out, pronto, so I kept quiet.

Mr P held my hand but looked over the blue curtain hanging between us and Dr Marcus and his team. I thought I may feel some rummaging around, but in truth I felt nothing. Mr P later said he would never tell me what they did to me, he was in truth fascinated by it all. A year later he had totally forgotten all the details. So, I will never know.

Then Elbo was out and on a table, being assessed for his Apgar score, which if I remember correctly was a healthy eight and I heard Mr P joke, *'blue eyes, big feet, white skin. I need to talk to my wife.'* Mr P is of Indian origin. I was too wasted to warrant that with a response. In fact, throughout the whole process, I think everyone had expected the air to be blue and I had stayed almost silent.

Then there was baby Elbo in front of me, wrapped in a towel. All I could see was a triangle shaped part of his face. He was OKAY, he was more than okay, he was beautiful, but most of all he was safe and healthy. The relief was intense.

Then I closed my eyes. I could hear everyone as Dr Marcus stitched me up, Mr P and the girls were joking, the atmosphere palpably lighter but I was wrecked, I could not muster any energy to do anything except lie there and breathe and feel such gratitude and solace in what had been a long roller coaster.

With hindsight, weeks later I recalled during pregnancy I had done a candle meditation after a prenatal yoga class and seen a triangular shaped baby's face in my third eye, my baby's face. Obviously, it was a sign. Hindsight is a marvellous tool and the universe is showing us signs all the time, if we can just be open to receiving them.

In recovery they tried to give me my baby to hold but my arms were like jelly, they felt as long as Mr Tickle's but completely useless. I had no control of them so I refused, I was scared I would drop him. It was two hours later when I felt up to holding and feeding him. It was a long two hours. Actually, it had been a long two nights and almost three days.

Later that night, back in our room, desperate at last for some sleep, a nurse came in to help me up, telling me I had to walk around. I complied and an enormous outpouring of blood ended up on the floor.... this time I really did think it was my uterus making a break for it. No, she reassured me it's normal. Normal? That is not normal I thought.

Finally, I was allowed back to bed, by this time it was almost 1.00am. Suddenly, the lights went on and a porter entered in to clean up the mess.

'No thank you, do it in the morning, shukraan,' I probably shouted...I mean, what did a new mum have to do to get a much-needed night's sleep? By now my British politeness had evaporated.

'Okay madam' he replied, retreating as he switched off the lights and I heard the door close. At last, I thought, sleep.

Then I heard the hinges go and the sound of a mop scraping on the edge of the door as, bless him, he tried to clean up in the dark from behind the door. 'I can still hear you, go away,' I muttered.

The following morning Lizzie, one of our midwives, who the day before had noticed something was up, had called Dr Marcus (from inside a toilet so as not at alarm us), who came in to see me. She told me they had checked the oxygen levels in Elbo's blood and they were right at the point of being a whole different ball game. Had she not acted when she did and the team not acted so quickly and efficiently to safely deliver our baby boy, we may have been dealing with a very different scenario.

'I'm just telling you because I know this is not what you wanted, I know you wanted no intervention and a natural birth but I just wanted you to know it was the right decision.'

I looked at Elbo in his little cot and nodded at her, 'Lizzie, I know, I know it was the right thing, honestly, I am totally happy with the decision you guys made. At the end of the day all I wanted was him safe and healthy and he is, thank you so much.'

I will never ever forget Lizzie. We now live on opposite sides of the world and she has kids of her own now. If those three girls had not decided to be there for us during their Christmas holidays, things may have been so different. Many of the nurses in Kuwait are Filipino or Indian and not used to standing up to their Middle Eastern patients, who expect a certain level of subservience. Many of them may have waited just a bit too long to see if they could have had the birth I requested on my birthing plan instead of making the call, like Lizzie did. Imagine if I had not changed doctors and we had stayed with Dr Liability? Elbo may not be the glorious, healthy, vibrant, kind, gentle, amazing nine-year-old he is today.

So, what is my advice to you? Have a birthing plan, of course, it gives a sense of being marginally in control in a situation when really you are not. But be prepared to throw that plan out of the window, because often it doesn't go to plan and all that really matters is there is a happy healthy baby and mum. Drugs, no drugs, it is all a matter of taste. But no one's issuing medals at the end of the day.

And my other bit of advice? When you are gazing lovingly at your sweet baby sleeping soundly in their little Perspex cot, cherish those moments, don't for goodness sake do what I did, which was to look at him and think, '*this motherhood thing is going to be walk in the park, look at him, so peaceful and quiet, I'm going to get SO much done...*' because karma will bite you in the bum for such smug thoughts. But that is a whole different story.

And just in case you were wondering, we didn't actually call him Elbo.

My UK Birthing Story

After my first child, when I didn't even know I was pregnant until he was ten weeks, every subsequent pregnancy I knew almost immediately, within the first week or so. I now knew what to look for: no sore boobs or queasiness for me; instead I went off my morning coffee and my evening vino. Sure fire signs every time.

Unfortunately, I lost both of the next two babies. Both at six weeks when they were barely larger than my little finger nail. The first time, we had literally landed in Istanbul to begin our new life there. I spent the first evening in hospital being told there was no heartbeat, which I found incredibly hard to accept. How could you even find a heartbeat in something that wasn't even the size of my finger nail? After three doctors explained the same thing, I had no choice but to accept the sorry news.

Nine months later it was the same story. This time I feared the worse as soon as I saw the scan and clocked it was absolutely no larger than the last one. The first miscarriage I could accept: I reasoned that a lot of women unfortunately go through the same dreadful experience; it's nature's way of ensuring healthy offspring. Two meant it was a pattern.

The next pregnancy I vowed it was the last, I could not take the emotional turmoil of losing another baby. This time we were blessed. Monitored closely from the off, I was put on aspirin, some kind of hormones and a course of folic acid. No swimming, no exercise, and definitely no s*x. I am not sure if this is just a Turkish thing or regular advice. By thirteen weeks I was elated, we had made it past the heart beat phase and even to the date most acknowledge the pregnancy to be safe and announcable.

I'm a talker and had talked about all my miscarriages from the offset. I feel sad regarding the taboo surrounding miscarriages. Of course, you don't necessarily want to be telling the postman and then potentially having to share the awful news if something goes wrong, but surely such horrible news you would want to share with your best friend or mum? But like I say, I am a talker, I pretty much talk my way into, through and out of everything, it is my processing tool.

So, by thirteen weeks I was ready to high-five the doc, unfortunately not the lovely Dr Marcus, who was still in Kuwait, but a lovely lady, whose name I can no longer remember, such is baby-brain. But she held my high-fiving and raised it, '*at sixteen weeks we will know you are having this baby,*' she stressed. Another three weeks wait.

Then Mr P announced that since Downs Syndrome ran in his family, (an elderly aunt had it), he wanted an amniocentesis, well not him personally, he wanted me to have one. Cue a series of difficult conversations, or what is technically known as full-blown marital disputes. I knew I could not live with myself if our healthy baby became another statistic due to a failed amniocentesis, however, on the other end of the scale, I knew he could not live with it if we did not do it and had a baby with Downs. It is not a feeling I understand or support to be honest. I know I would love and support any child we had regardless of their difficulties. He felt very differently. Adamantly differently, so at seventeen weeks we had the amnio.

Actually, it was an interesting experience. I watched it all. The doctor waited until our baby was way on the other side of my womb, inserted an enormous needle which you could see on screen going into my belly, extracted the liquid, which looked like pee, ('*well essentially that's what it is,*' summed up the doc) and the horrible ordeal was over pretty quickly and painlessly.

The wait for the results, a week, was not so quick or painless. Of course, every scenario goes through your mind but the doctor had said the whole procedure could not have gone better and not to worry, so that's what I tried to do: not worry.

We were delighted to get the results: no abnormalities and no adverse effects of the amnio on the baby. Hurrah, hurrah and a million times hurrah.

Nowadays, in just a few short years, there is a blood test which can confirm birth abnormalities, the baby's sex, lots of very cool and interesting stuff, without the need for this ordeal.

Two weeks later we found out we were having a girl, which was a huge shock; I honestly thought I could not carry girls, which is why I had had two miscarriages and that of course this baby was a boy. I then had a couple of weeks of selfishly feeling disappointed. I was afraid of having a girl, I could cope with a boy, but a girl, all that drama, all those moods, all that teenage angst, err no thanks. When I finally '*fessed up'* to Mr P about my feelings, he, in his usual down to earth fashion, dismissed it with, '*well that is a bloody load of bloody bollocks.*' And all my fears evaporated with his touchy feely twenty first century man-ness.

We chose a name, Indie. Meg, which was the name we had chosen for Akiro when we thought he was a girl, no longer worked. Funny how important a name was a few years previously and suddenly it was redundant.

Our parenting instinct, or lack of, is legendary. We were so convinced Akiro was a girl, that we joked if he was a boy we would call him Elbo. He was nicknamed Elbo for the whole of the second half of my pregnancy and well into the first few days of his life.

So, I was having a girl, we had her name picked out, her big brother was beside himself with...actually I don't know what...twenty weeks is a very long wait for a not quite three-year-old, so he was probably bemused and excited and frustrated, along with lots of other feelings he neither knew how to express, nor what they were.

Then it became apparent that my husband's two-year contract was up in November. It was always very likely it was only going to be a two-year gig and he was already exploring the next opportunity we would be thrust into: we know we are having this baby girl, we just don't know where.

As the end date arrived and no definite decision on the next job or location had been decided upon, we packed up all our stuff into storage and went to Goa for three weeks. We have an apartment there and it was a glorious three weeks of sunshine and relaxation. We even investigated a hospital to have Indie but at the ninth hour, with Christmas looming and people expecting us for the festivities, combined with an awareness of the limitations it would thrust upon our daughter if she were born outside of the UK, which we had already unwittingly lumbered our son with, (namely he must marry and have his kids in the UK for them to be liable for full British Citizenship), and my final fit to fly date looming, we headed back to Turkey to pick up our baby stuff and then head onto the UK.

Except, having been signed off fit to fly the day before our flight, the night before we left, deciding to play safe and eat pizza instead of Indian food to avoid any last-minute tummy upsets, what did I get? Food poisoning. It started just before we got in the taxi to the airport and continued for several hours. I nearly redecorated some unsuspecting people when they came out of the arrivals hall as I vomited over the wall when we arrived outside departures.

As I sat under a fan in Goa airport, looking anything but fit to fly, Mr P convinced the airline staff to check me in. As I boarded the plane, green around the gills, almost all the other passengers handed me their sick bags and the pilot came to greet me. We explained I was running out of days to fly and he allowed us on board.

In Turkey, we ended up sleeping on a friend's sofa as by the time we arrived there, Heathrow has been closed due to snow. Mr P spent almost twenty-four hours at Ataturk airport finally getting us on the first plane out of Istanbul into London. It was with enormous disappointment therefore, when we landed and looked out of the window, expecting to see snow ploughs, undulating snow drifts glistening in the moonlight, the odd yeti bounding across the scenery to see...well nothing except a bit of grey, sloppy, sludge. 'Mummy, where is the snow?' asked Akiro. Good point well made, little man. Once again, the UK transportation system was drowning under, well not that unusual weather.

Christmas came and went and we moved into the outlaws, as I affectionately call Mr P's parents. They have always maintained a larger house than they need in case any of their eight offspring find themselves as we were, homeless and in need of a roof over our heads. I had objected over the suggestion, as nobody with a new-born baby needs to be staying with relatives of any kind in my view. But beggars can't be choosers, was Mr P's view, so there we were.

Our first appointment with the family doctor was not encouraging. After a successful, but relatively frightening emergency C-section with my first born, I was all set for an elected C-section. Mostly because I did not want a repeat of the first time: three days of labour and emergency surgery. Also, because, I already had the sunroof, why couldn't she come out of that and maintain the integrity of the other exit option, to put it somewhat bluntly. Who needs or wants a wizard's sleeve and a sunroof?

The family's GP had other ideas. '*You won't get an elected C-section here.*' He professed and in the spirit of doom and gloom continued suggesting it wise not to admit we had been in Turkey because they would charge us for having the baby in the UK, so don't divulge my pregnancy notes to the midwife.

What? I was horrified. So, it's perfectly okay for anyone from within the EU to pop to the UK for free NHS treatment. But a bona fide UK citizen who had lived outside of the UK for the previous few years could not. After consulting another midwife friend of ours, (we have an awful lot of midwives in our friendship circle I have to admit), she was as horrified as I was and urged us to of course share our notes since, especially being so far along, if we did not, we would probably have social services on our doorstep. Seriously, why can nothing be simple? Well if it was, I would obviously be bored stupid and have nothing to wax lyrical about, so such is life.

Of course, an elected C-section is a different kettle of fish from an emergency one. We were urged not to do it by the doctor we met with to set a date, who stressed, 'this birth could be a whole different experience than the last one.' 'Or not,' I countered, 'and it was terrifying and I do not want to go through that experience again. Anyway,' I continued, 'Akiro needs someone to look after him while I am having this one,' I nodded at my son and rubbed my bump for dramatic effect, 'And...' I was on a roll now, 'my husband's parents are in their late eighties, they can't look after Akiro, I need to know what is happening and when, so that I can plan things for him.'

A list of things that could go wrong were detailed to me. Again, I countered this list saying, 'I never heard of any of these when it was an emergency and since we did not encounter any of them then, I am going with the hope we won't this time. Shall we set a date?' So, we did. 15th February. Both my kids it seems were to be the day after an *important day* kind of kids.

As the date neared, helpful passers-by would ask my due date and nod discouragingly, proclaiming I was carrying very low, *'you won't get that far'* and I was beginning to regret our decision to return to the UK, when did people get so doom and gloom about everything?

We renovated the room we were all to sleep in since although the outlaw's house is indeed large, the layout is odd and there was no logical solution to sleeping arrangements except for us to all share one room together. We cleared the room, painted the walls, laid carpet and installed three beds and the cot. All very happy families.

Meanwhile, every morning, I forced soggy Weetabix down while Ba, my mother-in-law slurped her chai from the saucer (and there were actual real mugs in the cupboards, it still bemuses me), and dada, my father in law, recooked yesterday's chapatti's in burnt butter. It was a sensory over-load even for the un-end of term observer, for me, all raging hormones and ready to pop, it was all a bit much.

Finally, Valentine's Day arrived and we delivered Akiro to Grandma Jacq's, my mum's. She had agreed to look after him overnight as I was required to be at the hospital the following morning at 6.00am. We settled him in and returned to Leicester for a very non-Valentine's evening, sharing the sofa with Mr P's brother while we scoffed a Sainsbury's ready meal and watched *'127 Hours'* about the mountain climber who got stuck under a bolder, all very romantic, not.

The next morning, up and at the hospital early doors, we were ready to go. We were not the first ones in but we didn't wait long. As they inserted the epidural they advised me I had scoliosis. My father had severe scoliosis and this is the first time anyone had ever noticed it in me. I can only assume all those years of a baby and toddler on my hip had warped my spine. It had warped my mind, so why not my spine?

Mr P was keen to watch over proceedings as he had in Kuwait, but the nursing staff had other ideas and reprimanded him telling him this was not about him. Touche McFly. Suddenly everything was interrupted and we were advised that the doctor had had to go out to deal with an emergency but not to worry, we were at a stage where I was fine to be put on hold.

Well, it is what it is, but no sooner had they had explained this, the doc was back and we were good to go. I had explained that I believed I was sensitive to the epidural since with Akiro's birth, I could not feel a thing and had lost the use of my arms. Whether they went easy on the drugs or because I was not even in labour, whatever the reason, I was fully aware of the pushing, prodding and tugging involved in getting little Indie out. There was a good deal of rummaging going on, that's for sure. And then she was out and in our arms. She still loves to this day, finding that first photo and asks every time, '*why did you and Daddy have that funny blue hat on, mummy?*'

It was a completely different scenario to Akiro's birth. I remember all the small details and the general chit chat on the operating table and the very light-hearted atmosphere, which was a stark contrast to the serious, down to business efficiency and speed which culminated the final minutes of Akiro's birth. I could also hold her straight away because my arms were working and so there was no delay in the new-born cuddles, which was a huge relief.

I had requested a private room. After my 5-star experience in Kuwait, a hospital ward was not for me. Not in a snobbish way, but because I knew no one in Leicester and my mum had already refused to bring Akiro to visit us the afternoon Indie was born, saying her car was not up to the journey. There is a lot of background to this that I won't bother to explain here but suffice to say, I did not wish to be publicly humiliated as the only person on the ward without visitors. My privacy in these crucial first few hours together was paramount. Again, this was very different from Kuwait, where we had streams of visitors every day.

Mr P headed off soon after lunch to pick up Akiro. Unfortunately, they did not make it back in time for visiting hours that day so we all had to wait until the next day to be reunited and for the siblings to meet each other. It was the Brit awards that night so Indie and I enjoyed our first night together watching that.

Her little Perspex cot was not at the end of my bed like in Kuwait it was next to the bed. The little private room was so tiny that every time anyone came in, the door bashed into the little crib. By the time we left, whenever the door hinges creaked, Indie startled before the door even crashed into her bed.

The staff were amazing, I felt cared for and supported. It wasn't 5-star luxury in surroundings but it was first rate care. I did of course miss Lizzie and Dr Marcus being on hand; I didn't even know the names of any of my doctors or nurses and despite reservations about returning to the outlaws, I was keen to get back to our humble bedroom with all four of us together. The reassurance waking up at night to hear everyone's breathing, without having to get up and check on them was a real delight.

We ended up staying for nearly six months. Many moments were heart-warming and delightful during that time: especially the bond Ba had with Indie, wrapping her in her sari and soothing her when she cried; watching Bollywood movies with her grandparents and there are many elements of our stay that left a lasting legacy, for better or for worse. But again, that is another story.

Alex Bannard's Biography

A modern-day nomad, Alex has travelled extensively and lived in Kuwait and Bangkok, Istanbul and Bavaria with her young family. A yoga and mindfulness teacher, she delves into that adventure called life and waxes lyrical about all aspects of living abroad, being a mum and anything else that inspires her. She is currently completing a book, chronicling her own experiences with post-natal depression and the arduous, but sometimes amusing, journey of recovery, in the hope it may help others in a similar position.

Glo Butane

I had a completely natural water birth in the end (main-part) without pain relief. I started out intending to have pain relief in the water birth part, (main/second part) but in the end, I forgot to ask for it because they had put an intravenous cannula in my left wrist, in case there were bleeding problems and told me to keep it out of the water; it was put in wrong and hurt so much that I was concentrating so hard on it and keeping it dry, I think it took my mind off the labour pain. I am surprised I made it without pain relief but I think ironically the pain from the cannula helped me focus (the crowning was the worst).

My contractions started Wednesday afternoon around 4.30pm but we didn't go into hospital until 1.00am on the Thursday. They said I wasn't dilated enough but kept me in. I was so tired from everything I finally asked for the pethidine injection in first stage, (amazing I loved it, it helped me rest a little bit and dilate and although I could still feel the contractions, I could rest in between). Finally, they came back to me at around 6.30am when the pethidine had already worn off for a while (and sometime during this time my waters finally broke). They set up the birthing pool and the cannula and the baby was finally born at 8.59am. Then, the afterbirth part, (the third stage), I remembered to ask for gas and air and amazingly, they told me I didn't receive any tears, so luckily there were no stitches, but I really think this was down to all the raspberry leaf I was taking (pills and tea) for at least a month before.

It was very surreal when the baby came out of me into the water, because he came out with his eyes wide open and blinked and then stared at me.

My husband said that it looked like a coconut with black hair was coming out and then the head turned and he saw eyes looking back.

But the strangest thing was when I was in my teens, (when my menstrual cycle first started), I was told by doctors and a gynaecologist that it was very unlikely that I would ever be able to have a natural birth because of the shape of my womb, (it's tilted), and the size of my hips. But luckily my husband and I met a really amazing midwife in antenatal class who mentioned many homeopathic remedies, birthing tips etc. so I have a few tips there which I think helped prepare me and also for the recovery. But not everyone is so lucky, as no matter how much you plan for the day, it is bound to take its own path.

Glo Butane's Biography

Glo is a musician, actress, and entrepreneur. She has also launched her own beauty business, *'Secrets of Glo'*.

My Birth Experiences by Paola Bagnall

I have two sons, now aged forty-two and forty. When I gave birth, things were very different to what they are now!

I think I was in natural hypnosis on both occasions, as I was so excited and both were natural births. I had wanted a baby since I was ten years old.

I had a good first pregnancy. I put on two and a half stone due to lots of amniotic fluid. I felt in a very holy state. My baby was very active and when he kicked in the last weeks you could see his entire foot sticking out of my tummy!

My first son was two weeks overdue and I had my waters broken in hospital at 9.30am, as there were no pessaries or drips back then of synthetic oxytocin. He was so ready to be born that I had a very short latent stage of labour and went almost immediately into the active stage with very strong contractions coming very quickly. Everything progressed very easily and I felt very lucky. In those days you were given pethidine almost automatically and I did not question this at the time. I had the most amazing hallucinations and during the time it had the effect that I lost control a bit. I refused any more. I had a transition period as I was ready to push but my cervix was not fully dilated. This was the most painful time but fully bearable. When I was able to push, the contractions became completely pain free. I had read this in the book '*The Natural Childbirth*', by Erna Wright and I was amazed to find it was true, as I was so focused on getting the baby out to see him. I was given an episiotomy, which was standard procedure all those years ago but I did not feel it at all. For the birth I was positioned on my side, the new idea then! I remember feeling sad as I could not see my baby being born.

My baby arrived just six hours after induction; I was thrilled he was a boy – no scans then to know the sex. I recall the joy of holding him, that magical moment where bonding seems to become so intense. I felt complete, as I really wanted to be a mother. I turned to my husband and said, "*well, I can go through that three more times*" as I had planned four babies!!

This to me was a perfect experience and the feeling of that first contraction was the most incredible moment of my life, probably because I am a biologist and I was so enthusiastic to know what it felt like! I found the entire process an exhilarating and empowering one. A great feeling!

My second pregnancy was a very different experience. I had nausea for four months, only put on one and a half stone and carried the baby differently, probably because the baby was in a slightly different position. As his feet were so close to my bladder in the last few weeks, when he kicked I wet myself!!

Twenty-two months after my first son, my second baby was born. This birth was not quite so short.

We were not checked as regularly then, as you are now and I was allowed to go three weeks overdue, even though I seemed to be two centimetres dilated with no contractions when my GP examined me at the weekly check-up. He was surprised I had not been feeling any contractions. I left my first child in bed asleep and went into hospital late at night ready to be induced in the morning. I started having very mild contractions around midnight so things had begun. They decided to break my waters in any case to speed things up for me, but this proved impossible as the amniotic sac was stuck to the baby. I had been wetting myself, and being a biologist I knew I was leaking amniotic fluid. I had told my GP this and he was not too bothered.   It turns out I had leaked most of the surrounding baby fluid and thus I had a dry birth which was like pushing a large tube of sandpaper out!! Still bearable, but the pushing stage was not totally pain free as before. In the end they used a special curved instrument to go around the baby's head to cut the membrane away from the baby so it could come out more easily. Baby was born about seven hours later and this time delivery was on my back and I was given the standard epidural. I have to admit that I had wanted a girl this time. Everyone had told me I was having a female as I was carrying so differently and the pregnancy was so very unlike the first one. However, I soon bonded with my red-haired baby and I am very happy with both my sons.

Again, the birth was a marvellous experience.

The female body is incredibly well designed to give birth. For me, the key factors for both births were being relaxed and in control, to let the body do what it needed to do. During those intense feelings of the contractions I found there was immense joy and pleasure as well.

Paola Bagnall's Biography

Paola is an experienced hypnotherapist who uses EFT (Emotional Freedom Technique) and Reiki in her work. She has a degree in biology and is a qualified teacher, with over thirty-five years' experience, first in a comprehensive school and then in a sixth-form college. She retired from teaching in July 2004 to take up hypnotherapy full-time, having set up her business *'Inner Power'* in 2000. She retired in 2015 from seeing clients.

Paola first learned self-hypnosis and found that she was able to tap into the inner power of the unconscious mind to heal a shoulder injury she had had for several years.   The medical profession had been unable to help her. Having discovered the innate ability we all have, to heal ourselves if we desire to, by harnessing these inner resources, Paola went on to become a fully qualified hypnotherapist, helping people to control pain and to heal themselves.

With her knowledge of biology and hypnotherapy, Inner Power Hypnobirthing was born! Hypnobirthing helps mothers to enjoy a wonderfully natural pregnancy and childbirth where the mum is in control.   With so many hypnobirthing success stories, Paola was persuaded to publish a book, *'Birth Made Easy'*, in 2011 on her unique method. In 2014 she launched an Application with the same name.

Paola used to run hypnobirthing workshops for the mums-to-be and their partners, and self-hypnosis workshops, teaching people how to use hypnosis to achieve their full potential.   She has trained many hypnotherapists in the Inner Power Hypnobirthing techniques (CPD workshops). In 2007, she ran a workshop on '*The Use of Hypnosis with Children'* in Albany, New Zealand.   In 2014, she gave a presentation on Inner Power Hypnobirthing at the HypnoThoughts Live Hypnosis Conference in Las Vegas, America.

Inner Power Hypnobirthing

Websites: http://www.innerpowerhypnobirthing.co.uk/
             http://www.birthmadeeasy.co.uk/
App link   http://hypnosisappstore.com/hypnobirthing/

Email: paola@innerpowerhypnobirthing.co.uk

Telephone: 020 8660 6022
Address: 40 Cliff End
             Purley
             Surrey
             CR8 1BN
             England

N D Hardwick

"Paracetamol My Dear?"

My first experience of child birth was unexpected to say the least. I had gone fourteen days over my due date, which is probably not all that unusual for first babies, but I was getting a bit 'antsy' to say the least! I had a bit of a scare with *placenta previa* towards the end of my pregnancy, where I was rushed into hospital and given steroids, but luckily it had moved around at the last moment so I could go ahead with a natural birth.

They admitted me to the maternity wing to be induced, to move things along a bit. By this time, as you can imagine, I was more than ready. I went in at 9.00pm, by the time I had been examined and given the induction gel it was almost midnight. The midwife said it was extremely unlikely anything would happen tonight, so she recommended my husband go home and return early in the morning.

Although reluctant, my husband left and I was all alone in this darkened room. I felt like I needed to go to the toilet. I had suffered from bad constipation and haemorrhoids throughout my pregnancy and passing was not a pleasant experience. I found myself in the toilet for a VERY-LONG-TIME pushing and eventually managed to pass something, but afterwards I still had cramps. I mentioned this to the midwife who basically said this was normal after taking the gel and not to worry as my waters hadn't even broken yet. She kindly offered, *"can I get you some paracetamol dear?"*

Of course, this being my first pregnancy I had no idea whether these cramps I was experiencing was just a bit of tummy ache or actual labour. I did explain to the midwife they were quite painful, but she didn't seem concerned and said it would probably be ages yet.

I couldn't help thinking that maybe my husband should be called, bearing in mind the hospital was a forty-five-minute drive away from our home, but decided to take the advice of the professionals and not panic just yet.

The midwife comes back with the paracetamol, which frankly I took, but did not think they would make an iota of difference to this excruciating pain I was experiencing. *"I'll get the birthing ball dear, might help move things along"* … I tried to sit on this thing but it was just too painful. The midwife still kept saying that inductions always take several hours so not to worry, it wouldn't be imminent. She left me alone.

With hindsight I should have insisted they call my husband, but I was totally ignorant to the whole process and trusted those people who had been doing the job for years.

Then it happened!!!! My waters broke…. It was quite a shock, I had just got off that darn ball thing and the balloon burst!   I pressed the call button and then the contractions really kicked in hard! The midwife came rushing in, *"now, you're going to tell me your waters have broken aren't you…oh….I can't believe it!   This has never happened so quick before."*

Well it has now lady!!!!!   At this point they checked me and I was almost fully dilated. It had all happened so quickly, they rushed me down to the delivery suite.   I remember screaming down the corridor to the lift and one of the staff shushing me… Hilarious! There was no shushing me!!

Once in the delivery suite, they told me my husband had been called, bless him…he made it in thirty minutes! He said, when he was ushered into the ward, the midwife told him, *"your wife is the one you can hear screaming at the end of the corridor"*. Well I have never exactly been a shrinking violet and childbirth was not an exception!

In the end, all I had was gas and air as that's all I had time for!   My son was born at 5.00am, so I was only actually in active labour for about two to three hours, thank the lord for small mercies!

I did feel rather spaced out once the birth was over, my hubby held our son while they stitched me up and rallied round me. When I held him, it really was a bit surreal; I don't know whether that was due to the gas and air, or just the overwhelming experience.

Although my birth was short, it was a totally mind-blowing experience, and it is true what they say, that there's never one the same.

My biggest labour tip would be: Expect the unexpected and you'll be just fine.

N D Hardwick's Biography

Current Status: Full time mother of two, lives in Grantham, Lincolnshire, UK

Mummy Blogger: *www.mumthemagician.com*   writing about all things related to Mummy Magic!

Education: Studied BSc Law with Management at the University of London.

Previous Profession: Business Analyst and IT Project Manager.

Debut Novel released January 2017: **A Devil Lies on My Shoulder**. A Supernatural thriller touching on very raw, real life issues of teenage angst; sexual discovery and abuse; criminal intent; emotional torment; family dynamics and of course the all-important element of sly, sometimes dark, humour.

Download on Kindle or buy paperback version on Amazon:

https://read.amazon.co.uk/kp/embed?asin=B01N5TRKMV&preview=newtab&linkCode=kpe&ref_=cm_sw_r_kb_dp_SXbRyb97GX7PP

My Birth Story
by Rachel Braun: Audrey

Warning! This may be a little long, but it did take FOREVER for this little girl to grace us with her presence. And she was worth every bit of agony I went through.

My due date was November 12th, 2003. From the very beginning of my pregnancy, knowing my due date, I had hoped my first baby would share her birthday with my Dad's birthday, November 14th. So, I never got that "*itchy*" feeling as I neared the end. I was so hopeful, that as the 14th came, I began to feel contractions. Since this was going to be the first grandbaby in my family and everyone was very excited, I called them.

They all showed up, (my sisters, my brother, my parents) and proceeded to watch me closely for two days straight. With bated breath, ready to rush to the hospital at any moment. I tried everything I could think of over that weekend to get labour going. I have never felt more like a zoo animal in my entire life. But things did not go as I had hoped, and everyone headed home to Milwaukee. It was at that point I should have realized this kid had her own plan.

I should preface this by saying that my goal was to have no unnecessary medical interventions during my pregnancy or labour. My husband and I had spent twelve weeks in Bradley classes, diligently preparing to have a natural childbirth. We were equipped with our two-page birth plan detailing everything the nurses, midwives, and doctors needed to know once we arrived at the hospital. I am certain they appreciated my instructions. And with most people telling me I was crazy and would never be able to do it, I was more determined than ever.

Needless to say, I did not want to be induced, and over the course of the next week, I once again tried every trick in the book to get labour going. Unfortunately, nothing worked. As the following weekend approached, now nine days overdue, I was scheduled to be monitored just to make sure the baby was still doing okay. I was having some contractions that Friday morning, and I decided that at my appointment, I would ask the midwife to strip my membranes in the hopes that it would help things along.

Since I was contracting, I was told to meet the midwife at the hospital so I could have my appointment in triage (just in case). I was put on the monitor and checked. Baby looked good, I was almost completely effaced, but I was barely beginning to dilate. It was confirmed that I was most likely in the very early stages of labour. The midwife agreed to strip my membranes, and then sent me home.

On the walk to the parking ramp, my contractions began to increase in intensity, though they were still too irregular and too far apart. Besides, I was resolved to labour at home as long as possible to avoid any embarrassing send homes from triage. The next time I was sent home from the hospital it would be with a baby in my arms.

On the way home, I stopped off at Walgreens to purchase a bottle of castor oil. This would be my *"last case scenario"* effort to induce labour if things did not proceed quick enough. I did not want to drink it, but I would if necessary.

My contractions continued throughout the day, but they still weren't painful enough to warrant action. I was trying to stay on my feet as much as possible; going for walks, vacuuming and cleaning the house, in order to keep labour progressing. As the evening approached, my contractions became more uncomfortable. I was having to stop and breath through them. So, around 10.00pm we made a trip back to triage.

With bags in hand, I was sure I would be staying this time. I was checked, and was only dilated by 2-3cm. I was told to walk the halls for an hour or so, and come back for a recheck. I walked and walked and walked, but when I was rechecked, I had not changed enough to be admitted. Much to my dismay, I was once again sent home.

I did not sleep a wink from Friday into Saturday. My contractions were much stronger at this point. I was doing a lot of leaning on walls and swaying. I even tried a bath to relieve the pain. After eight to ten hours of pretty regular, painful contracting, I finally decided to head back to triage Saturday morning. Just my husband and I this time, since we didn't want to bother anymore people with needless trips.

At last I was worthy of admission! Though I was a little disappointed to hear that after all those hours of contractions, I was still only 4cm dilated. Once I was settled in my room, we made the calls to family. This time they could come; we had been admitted. There would finally be a baby at some point.

After a couple of hours of labouring in the hospital, I was checked again. Not much progress. At this point, we discussed breaking my water to move things along. My husband and I decided this would be a minimally invasive intervention which could hopefully send me sailing towards birth. So, we did it.

Once my water was broken, it was apparent that meconium was present. I was now ten days overdue after all. This led to more interventions I had originally not wanted. Namely, continuous monitoring. I was strapped to a machine and basically confined to my room.

At this point, my memory gets a little jumbled. I had a lot of visitors throughout the day, since the entire family had returned to see this baby born. I was in a lot of pain, so the movies I brought to distract myself basically served no purpose. And every time I was checked, I became more frustrated because I was just barely progressing. The baby was occipital posterior, which means she was face-up, the opposite of optimal for delivery. It also means her skull was basically grinding against my lower back with every contraction.

Because of her position, she was not moving down fast enough. She was not putting enough pressure on my cervix to dilate it. And I was having horrible back pain. Just to relieve the pain slightly, my husband was having to put all his weight into pushing on my low back during contractions.

At some point in the evening, nearing twenty-four hours in labour, we agreed to a low level of Pitocin. We were hoping to make each contraction more productive, in doctor speak. It was also at this point, we decided to try an internal version. This is basically where the midwife puts her entire hand into my vaginal canal, and attempts to grab the baby's head in an effort to flip her into the correct position. Mind you, I had not had any pain meds at this point.

I was told to get on all fours on the top of the bed. My husband and one of the midwives held opposite ends of a bed sheet that was positioned cradling the base of my belly. They were told to pull up (basically to disengage the baby from my pelvis) while the other midwife reached in to turn her. No kidding, I still cringe when I think of this. To this day, this is the most painful thing I have ever experienced in my life. The entire birthing floor heard my scream. My family thought I was giving birth, the scream was so loud.

And despite my extreme efforts, the baby would not turn.

I was now reaching my limit. I was going on roughly thirty hours with no sleep. I was only 7cm dilated, I had just experienced the worst pain of my life, and I had no idea when the end would come. I needed to rest. The midwives feared that at the rate I was going, I would not have the energy to push once I reached that point. In addition, the baby's heart rate was beginning to concern the them.

Things were definitely not going according to plan. My husband and I discussed our options with the midwives. We decided it would be best to get an epidural. That way I could rest. They could increase the Pitocin, and hopefully by morning, I would be ready to deliver the baby.

The most difficult part of getting the epidural was having to stay completely still through my contractions. But it was worth it! Sweet, sweet relief! I could finally relax for a few hours. But without the pain to distract me, my emotions slammed into gear. The slight disappointment of things not going as planned combined with lack of sleep and anxiety about what was next, finally hit me. I will never forget the wonderful nurse that sat with me, listened to me cry, and gave me her words of encouragement. She definitely helped me get through the night.

When morning came, roughly 5.00 or 6.00am, I was rechecked and our prayers were answered; I was finally 10cm! It was time to push. The midwives decided it would be a good idea to turn the epidural down a bit so I could better feel the contractions. BIG MISTAKE! When the pain was incrementally increased over a long period of time, I was able to handle it. But take that extreme pain away for several hours, and then bring it back? No fucking way!!

After an argument with the anaesthesiologist, the epidural was increased. And after some instructions from the midwife and nurses, I was pushing effectively. Though, that also meant I emptied my bowels (much to my husband's dismay.) I pushed and pushed and pushed, for roughly four hours.

Although her head could be seen with each push, she was not coming out. The doctors thought she could use a little assistance. Plus, I had already been labouring for more than forty hours and pushing for four hours, and they were not sure how much more I, or the baby, could handle. They wanted to get her out as soon as possible.

We decided to try a vacuum assisted delivery. Once everything was set up, they attached they suction cup to her head, and with the next push, they pulled. The vacuum popped off. So, they tried again. And it popped off again.

At this point, I knew where we were heading. I had tried everything. I was tired. I was ready to meet my baby, and I was prepared to do what it took to get her out. I signed the consent for a caesarean section. I talked to my family, who had been waiting for nearly two days in the waiting room, and they reassured me. And with that, I was rolled towards the operating room.

Once in the O.R., things moved pretty quick. They got me prepped, and then it was time to test whether the epidural was sufficient for surgery. It was not. I could just barely feel the sharp prick on my abdomen. I needed to be put under. I would not be awake to see my baby born, and my husband had to leave the room as well. It seemed throughout this experience I could not catch a single break.

Of course, I do not remember anything past this point, though I am grateful for the video my midwife was able to get of the event. Yet, I do recall the first moments as I was coming out of anaesthesia. I distinctly heard someone say, "*It's a girl!*" I was beyond ecstatic. And when I was in recovery, and at long last got to hold my baby, it was all worth it.

Rachel Braun's Biography

Rachel Braun is a busy mother of four crazy kiddos, three girls and one boy, aged 5-13. When she is not frantically running around after her children, you can find her writing, swimming, biking, running, or eating everything in sight (hence the exercise). She enjoys helping other moms lead healthy, balanced lives through her blog at www.mywildjourney.com.

The Best Father's Day Present
by Motherhudds
34 weeks...

I remember this very well. I was brushing my teeth and my husband was staring at my bump affectionately.

"There's no way you are going to go full term, you are massive!" He said.

As I was pregnant this is the only way my husband would ever get away with saying the words "*you are massive*" and live.

He affectionately jiggled my belly and said night-night to the bump. Usually the baby would kick a bit in response, but this time I felt an almighty '*pop*' and got instant tummy ache.

Nothing happened immediately so I went to bed just thinking the baby had jolted and he must've woken her up, but when I woke up approximately three hours later, everything was wet.

The thing is, when you are pregnant, peeing yourself sort of comes with the territory. Sometimes you pee a little if you sneeze, cough, hiccup, laugh even. So even though I was drenched, my first thought when waking up was that I'd had an '*accident*' and that it had to happen sooner rather than later. However, when I got up, I realised that I was leaking. Everywhere. And not just a little bit, it was like someone had turned a tap on inside me.

My husband, who had been fast asleep up to that point, stirred and turning slowly towards me, he opened one sleepy eye and said "honey, do you know you are weeing on the carpet?"

After that it was a blur.

Once we had established that my waters had broken, my hubby flung everything into the back of the car and laid a towel over the front seat for me to leak on.

Whizzing through the deserted streets of Yorkshire at some ungodly hour, I was struggling to grasp the reality of what was going on. It was surreal. This wasn't the plan. This wasn't supposed to happen now; it was too early. A thousand questions flooded my brain, each one coming as fast as the one before it, piling on top of each other into a mound of sheer confusion. I couldn't process anything so instead I stared out of the window and watched the streetlights blur as we passed.

I'm not a fan of hospitals, I'm not going to lie, so I don't think the reality of what was going on truly hit me until we arrived. The carpark was deserted and we had to ring a small inconspicuous buzzer to get in. I remember the disembodied voice crackling out of the intercom asking why we were there at 3.00am and having a complete and utter moment of blankness as I mumbled something about me wetting myself and having a baby…..

Oh my. That's right, I was having a baby. I. Was. Having. A. Baby.

Me, the person who can't work the microwave properly and burns everything I cook. Me, the person who doesn't even know if we own an iron, let alone how to turn it on. Me, the person who leaves her £1 in the trolley slot pretty much every time we go to Sainsbury's. Me, who regularly walks into walls, doors and falls over pavements or my own feet. Me, who rarely makes it through a meal without spilling it on myself, the sofa and/or one of the cats. Me, the person who would never even make it to work without my husband dragging me out of bed and making me breakfast, as I have the ability to sleep through the apocalypse. Me. That person.

Wham. There it was, the big-smack-in-the-face reality of the situation. How the hell was I going to take care of a baby when I could barely take care of myself?

As I got in the lift to go to the maternity assessment unit, all I kept thinking was *'next time I get in the car the baby will be with us'* and *'next time I walk through my front door, we will have the baby with us'*. It was a weird, surreal, unimaginable moment in my life. These thoughts continued to swirl through my head clouding my faculties as I walked, leaving a small trail of water behind me.

After about eighteen years, I was finally examined by the specialist and about thirty-two other people who all had a good poke round down there, whilst the area was illuminated by a gigantic spotlight that would have been more at home in Wembley arena. All the while this was going on, the woman in the next bed to me, who was in labour, screamed like she was being tortured, whilst intermittently shouting through the curtain to me that *'it wasn't as bad as it sounds'.* Call me a sceptic, but she sounded like she was having her eyelids pulled over her ears and she kept threatening to strangle her husband with the gas and air cord.

After a good search, the conclusion from the specialist was that the indeed my waters had broken. I wanted to say: "No shit Sherlock, there's a frigging river beneath the bed", but what I actually said was *"oh, really?"*   I didn't feel I was in any position to be sarky with legs akimbo and Blackpool illuminations shining on me, whilst speaking to someone in a white coat holding a contraption that looked suspiciously like a car jack.

Eventually they hooked me up to a trace machine to monitor the baby and gave me a scan. Unfortunately, when they scanned me, they discovered the baby was breech. Because she was breech and my waters had gone, it was very unlikely they could turn her and so they weren't entirely sure what to do. In my hazy middle of the night muddled state, I vaguely recall them mentioning the words *'C-section'* to me but I was so tired at that point I was happy just to go to bed for a couple of hours or so and see what was happening in the morning. With any luck the baby will be here by then and I will have slept through the whole experience. Ha, ha, ha.

At about 5.00am, a bed was eventually located and I was led to the antenatal ward and introduced to what would be my home for the next few days. My '*home*' was shared with three other women in varying stages of their labour process, but all of whom, had some kind of issue from placenta previa to their waters breaking, like me.

After I'd had about thirty minutes sleep, I was woken up by the midwives. Due to some complications I'd had with Group B Strep, I was on antibiotics throughout my labour so after listening to the baby and checking my temperature and blood pressure, I was given my bout of antibiotics.

It's quite disorientating being in hospital where they work on a twenty-four-hour schedule, as you are never truly sure what time of the day or night it is, particularly as the rounds are done quite frequently. As an end result, you get very little sleep and end up feeling a little like you're hallucinating.

This does not work in harmony with having to make decisions and as an end result when the consultant came to see me in the morning to discuss my situation, instead of having a grown up intellectual level-leaded conversation, I burst out crying before she had opened her mouth and said I wanted my mum. Once calmed by a couple of midwives, the consultant, who clearly felt I was a neurotic inconvenience, told me that having analysed my results and situation, that the best plan of action for me would be a Caesarean section.

The world spun on its axis.

C-section? Major surgery?! I cry at a paper cut! How can I be cut open?!

They explained that I had very little amniotic fluid left and so it would be impossible for them to turn the baby from the breech position and as I am GBS positive, she was at risk of infection the longer she stayed inside me. I was given the choice; a C-section to take place as soon as possible when I could be fitted in – classed as a '*semi emergency C section*' and therefore my husband could be with me, or an emergency C-section, where they wait for me to go into labour and as soon as I do, they do the section, but for this I would be put to sleep and my husband could not be in with me. Seemed kind of a no-brainer, but I wanted to wait and discuss it with my hubby when he arrived at 8.00am so asked if I could be given a little more time. In fear of a repeat tantrum, and the threat of bringing in my mum in (she must know her), the consultant left me to it until he arrived.

Once he arrived I promptly burst into tears again and explained to him the best I could what the consultant had said between snotty sobs (mine, not consultant). I could see him go through an array of emotions as his brain processed the information and came to the realisation that our baby was going to be born early and his wife was going to undergo major surgery; neither of which sounded very good.

Everyone kept reassuring us that thirty-four weeks was a good gestation and she would do very well and that C-sections were perfectly safe. A reassurance I would have been happy to subscribe to had I not then been handed a consent form to sign that explained, in graphic detail and using big, long, important words, all number of horrible things that could happen to me or the baby during the procedure. In the end we went with the obvious choice and opted for the semi-emergency section and got my ticket in the queue.

C-sections nowadays are done on kind of a conveyer belt system where basically you wait your turn based on your needs and so there was a few women before me in the queue. In the meantime, my husband tried to entertain and distract me the best he could without showing the true extent of his concerns. He did well until he had to call my parents to inform them of the situation and broke down as soon as my dad answered the phone. As a general rule, my husband is very calm and not emotional. He's generally quite level headed and is a *'fixer upper'* of things and on the whole, where I would react like a three-year-old, he is the grown up. However, with everything going on all at once and then having to relay it all, it clearly got a bit much for him.

Of course, my parents, knowing how stable he generally is, completely freaked out hearing him upset and my dad just said, *"we are on our way,"* without much discussion at all.

In line with how my day was going, my emotional parents turned up just as I was dressed in my very fetching *'scrubs'* ready for my C-section, complete with full back gape which showed off my humongous knickers.

I must've looked a right sight to my parents as I stood there like a giant round blue ball in my fetching open backed gown, with my knee high anti-blood clot tights on, Disney slippers on and tears streaming down my face, as they had been for the last few hours. I may very well have been off to have a baby, but right at that very moment all my mum and dad saw was their own baby, very upset. Which in turn, upset them.

My dad, like my husband, is not a crier at all. I could count on one hand the times I've collectively seen the pair of them get emotional over anything, but I could see my dad found it distressing to see me upset, knowing I was going for a major operation and it's hard to see that. As a result, I got a massive parental bear hug as hubby held the back of my gown to save my dignity because he'd tied the ties wrong (should've known then it didn't bode well for a baby-grow).

Eventually I peeled myself away from my mum and dad and left them sat by my bed in the ward, whilst my husband and I shuffled down to the operating room, him behind me, holding my gown together. I don't know if it was just because of the situation I was in, but it felt like a long walk and it did nothing to help when we were asked to wait outside whilst the room was prepped.

I kept seeing a variety of people walk in and out of the swing doors, allowing me just a glimpse of the array of machinery and equipment in there and I can tell you now, that just piled the cherry on the cake of my anxiety. Once all the attire was correctly positioned and fastened we were summoned to the operating room and, as if she knew, the baby gave a big shudder; probably trying to hide in my rib cage somewhere as she sensed the dramatic entrance she was about to make.

I was helped up onto a higher than necessary bed; a feat not in any way dignified when your backside hangs out of an open gown and you are trying to lift a wiggling bump up onto it using what can only be described as a child's toilet step. An unsteady one at that.

Eventually I managed to get into position and two anaesthetists came to administer my epidural.

I will tell you now, that epidural hurt! Well, it was more the local anaesthetic that hurt the most as it's inserted into your spine, it's so stingy! Having an epidural has got to be one of the weirdest feelings I've ever had. You can literally feel the fluid flooding around your body and through your system until your lower half becomes completely immobile. To gauge your level of feeling the anaesthetists spray freezing cold spray onto various parts of your body to see what you can and can't feel. Once they are happy that you cannot feel anything lower down, then they go ahead with the section. I remember my lower half feeling like it weighed a ton and it's the most bizarre feeling for your brain to want to do something like move your foot, but your body is completely unable to carry out that task. It was only when I'd lost complete feeling that I first became acutely aware of my surroundings and the seriousness of the situation, as I lay there unable to move like a beached whale.

There were fourteen people in that room that day, including me and my husband. The room was huge and I was unable to see right to the edges of it. It was stark white, filled with beeping machines, wires and things that pulsed and pumped everywhere. Gleaming silver, sharp looking tools lay on a sterile tray, waiting for the surgeons to do their work, and in the corner stood two NICU staff with an incubator and oxygen waiting to take the baby as soon as she was born. Things suddenly felt very serious.

I glanced over at my husband and even though he looked like a weird smurf in his scrubs, it still didn't make me laugh but instead, just added to the bizarre scene all around me, to which a backdrop of pop music played out from the radio. It looked like Area 51.

To the other side of me sat one of the anaesthetists who would stay there the whole time staring at me, to watch for any signs of feeling or pain so he could quickly top up the epidural if need be.

Then, the surgeon came in and the atmosphere in the room shifted. You could tell straightaway that the surgeon had entered, as she had an air of authority and respect about her, and all the staff stood up a little straighter. Despite this, she seemed very friendly and explained that she would talk me through each part of the procedure so that we knew what was happening. I was asked if I was ready and despite my brain saying '*no*' I said, in a small voice, "*as ready as I'll ever be*" and with that the screen was erected and they began.

My sister-in-law had described having a C-section to me like '*someone washing up in your stomach*' and I could see what she meant. It's bizarre. You don't feel any pain, you just kind of feel movement inside you and feel everything swirling about. There's a tightness that sort of loosens off as they proceed, presumably this is when you are cut and your skin gives way, it's a strange, strange, peculiar feeling. At the same time as all this, I could feel the baby wiggling around as if to say "*what the hell is going on here then,*" but of course I had no power of movement and no ability to see, so I just kind of laid there and listened and felt.

The surgeon quite abruptly asked for the radio to be switched off so she could concentrate and I was grateful for that as '*Tragedy*' was playing and making me even more nervous.

Whilst she stuck to her promise to talk through each stage, she may as well of been speaking Swahili as I didn't understand any of it as it was all very medical. Besides, I was thoroughly distracted by the noises coming from my tummy; squishing and squelching and sucking and swirling. Then suddenly, I felt a large pop and a lot of pressure followed by an almighty squelch and what felt like a vacuum cleaner sucking my insides out before an almighty scream and my daughter popped out into the world, bottom first, at 3.16pm.

Two become three...

As soon as she was out, they immediately took her over to the NICU staff for examination. In the brief flash I got, I could see she was small, very small, but she had a good set of lungs on her. The area where she was being examined was far over the other side of the room, as far away from me as possible and my husband had shot over there after her to cut the cord; a task he later tells me is like hacking through sausage knots with blunt scissors.

I hadn't realised how weak I'd become as I was trying to shout over to them *"is she a girl?"* Just to make sure that a boy hadn't unexpectedly popped out of there, who would then be forced to dress in pink for twelve months and live in a bright pink bedroom. No one could hear me though and I must've shouted six or seven times before my husband came over and confirmed she was indeed a girl.

She was 4lbs 14oz at birth and after a brief bit of oxygen she was breathing well, unaided and she was brought over to us so my husband could hold his baby girl for the very first time.

It happened to be Father's Day that day and as he cuddled his little bundle, he quietly said to her, *"thank you for the best Father's Day present ever"*, and right there, right then, in that one moment, we both fell head over heels in love with this little, red, squishy, noisy creature in a way we both never thought possible.

As she was small, premature and at risk of Strep B, she had to be taken away from us pretty quickly to receive vital antibiotics and go on a feed tube, so sadly after about five minutes and a brief kiss, she was taken away to the Special Care Baby Unit (SCBU) for treatment. I was eventually taken into an empty recovery room where my very emotional parents were waiting for us and we were allowed some time to process the situation. My parents fired a whole series of questions at me, none of which I could make sense of or answer as all my thoughts had gone to the SCBU with my tiny brand-new daughter. Instead I sat there quietly, shaking and shivering as the anaesthetic slowly made its way out of my body.

Eventually, my parents left and I was wheeled back to my ward and allowed to recover, but not before all my other ward mates pounced on me wanting to know every detail, which wasn't ideal as I could barely move from the epidural and had a catheter in. It's very disconcerting talking to people when your urine bag is gradually filling up next to their legs.

After what seemed like an eternity, they eventually left and we were left alone to go over the events of the day and make some sense out of the whirlwind that had been our life for the past twenty-four hours.

It's amazing really, when you think about how much your life can change in such a small space of time. I was a different person to who I was this time yesterday and the dynamics of our family had switched forever. It's incredibly overwhelming. I think for a good few minutes, we must've just sat there looking at each other in silent disbelief that we were now parents and in charge of such a tiny, vulnerable little person; made even more surreal by the fact that the baby wasn't with us. It was almost like we'd dreamt it.

Personally, I felt strangely empty without my wriggling bump, but at the same time released from all the heaviness, uncomfortableness and bloating I'd felt over the past few months. I was acutely aware that I could feel parts of my body again that I hadn't felt in a long time and new parts that I would need to get used to. It was all very peculiar and just processing the chaos and events that had taken place left both of us quite speechless and unable to find the right words.

The one thing that we both do very well though is go into *plan of action* mode and so before long, we stopped trying to unravel the craziness of the past, I ate a triple Bounty and we started to come up with a plan forward.

We knew our daughter would be in the SCBU for some time and so it was important to both of us that she was with a member of her family for the maximum amount of time and ideally, only left when she was sleeping. I wanted her to know from the beginning that she was never alone and we were always there for her. Because of this, my husband didn't stay long with me and as soon as he was allowed into the SCBU, he left to be with her.

I was unable to move due to the epidural which was still wearing off, but I was promised that as soon as I was able to, I'd be helped into the shower and then wheeled to my daughter's ward so I could finally hold her.

After thirteen long hours, I finally got taken to the SCBU to properly meet my baby daughter.

Handing her to me, still attached to wires and tubes, the midwives gently placed her in my arms and I got to hold my baby girl for the very first time. I felt this electric shock of emotion flood into every single part of my body, this overwhelming rush expanding my heart and a feeling that I never wanted to let go of. Instinctively, she turned into me and nuzzled close as I stroked her head and breathed in her soft brand-new baby scent. Despite being on a noisy, busy ward, it felt like there was no one else in the room with us, just me and her.

She looked so tiny and so vulnerable that I wanted nothing more than to protect her. Protect her emotionally, physically and mentally. No matter whatever happened in my life or where the path would take us, I vowed to always be there for her, right by her side. Right there and then I knew I was now a mother and despite my previous doubts, I had never felt so sure of my ability to take care of and love my child.

You simply cannot put into words the rush you get for your children. It's got to be the most magical, amazing, confusing, bizarre, heart-warming and all-consuming feeling. It's almost too much to bear, but it's like once you become a parent, you suddenly develop a brand-new sense. Every feeling that your child has, you feel; every need that they have, you take care of; every success that they experience, it's like it's happening to you. You feel proud, prouder than you've ever felt that you made this tiny perfect person. All these fingers and toes, the eyes, the ears, the little puckered mouth, you grew that.

Wow. She was outside of my body now but she was never going to truly leave me. She'd changed my biochemical make-up and would stay with me forever.

It was a long, long three weeks for us toing and froing from the Special Care Unit. Many tears were shed as her condition went up and down, and every night when I had to leave her and do the forty-minute journey home without her it broke me. But finally, after what felt like a lifetime, we were allowed to take our little girl home and be a family.

Now my daughter is a normal, cheeky two-and-a-half-year-old who has no lasting effects from her dramatic entrance to the world. We have since been blessed with our gorgeous son and our wonderful family is now complete.

My Labour Tips Would Be:

- By all means do a birth plan but be flexible. Make it clear what you will accept and what won't, but try not to have every detail mapped out, things usually don't go the way you think.

- Pack your hospital bag early!

- Try and stay calm. Okay, I know this is tricky and possibly the eagled-eyed ones of you may have noticed, I didn't have contractions. But I did with my second child, for thirty-six hours straight, so I do know what it feels like. But the best thing you can do is try and stay calm, and breathe. You'll be amazed what breathing through them can do.

- Accept pain relief. Now, this isn't a blanket *'accept all'* pain relief tip, but do consider what pain relief you'd like. I personally didn't want gas and air as I don't like feeling woozy, but I had two epidurals and a bucket load of paracetamol.

- Ask questions. Never be afraid to ask what's happing. It's your baby and your body, you are entitled to know. I asked a lot of questions throughout my section and found people more than willing to explain things. Be clear and if you aren't happy with something, speak up.

- Be clear to your birth partner on what you need. Remember they're there for you and this is the one time it's fully okay to make it all about you. Plus, it stops your birth partner trying to guess and do the wrong thing, thus incurring pregnant labour wrath - make them part of the whole experience.

- After the baby arrives, take some time out to process the events and clear your mind. Take quiet time to bond with your child and do skin on skin as early as possible. Those first few hours are when you and your partner should spend quiet time with your baby before having visitors. This lets you gather your thoughts and allows your baby that time to get used to being outside your body.

Motherhuggs' Biography

I'm a West Yorkshire mummy and live with my husband, our two children and our four cats. I run the social media site, *'MotherHudds'* which is for mums in Huddersfield. https://twitter.com/motherhudds

My Birth Stories by Louise George

My two birth experiences were very different from each other. My eldest daughter, Jessica, was born in hospital with the help of forceps; my youngest, Sophie, in a birth pool at home. Although very different, both births were positive experiences.

Jessica's Birth

My eldest daughter Jessica was diagnosed with a complex heart condition when I was twenty weeks' pregnant, which resulted in her having surgery in the womb when I was twenty-eight weeks' pregnant. We had originally hoped for a home birth but, as Jessica would need medical intervention as soon as she was born, we accepted that a hospital birth was necessary. We knew that there was a risk she wouldn't survive my pregnancy and labour which made this an anxious time. However, it was also a joyful time too – we focused on enjoying my pregnancy, not knowing whether that would be all the time we would have with Jessica.

Jessica was due to be induced at thirty-nine weeks, but I had a feeling she wasn't going to wait until then! My instincts were right – a week before the induction date, I woke up at 4.00am with mild contractions. At 6.00am, with the contractions coming every eight minutes, I woke my husband up. He was due to set up a big event that day. His first reaction was *"Not today! I have an event to set up!"* followed by *"Well it's on the way to the hospital... maybe we could stop off on the way. Do you have any black clothes so that you'll blend in with the crew?"*

I'm not quite sure that I would have ever *"blended in with the crew"* at eight months' pregnant, but as I knew it was still early on labour-wise, I was happy to go along with this. I should probably add at this point that I worked as a midwife up until going on maternity leave to have Jessica and so I was very aware of what stage we would need to go to the hospital. I also knew that my husband was relying on me to tell him when we reached this stage!

My waters broke as we got ready to leave. Jessica was moving about and the fluid was clear so I was happy to continue with our plan and go on to the hospital as needed later on. The contractions were still mild and infrequent. As we took a last long look around the house, I prayed that we would have Jessica with us when we returned.

I was aware of every movement, feeling relieved that Jessica was being her usual active self. I was excited that things had started happening, but I was also scared. Soon we would be meeting our precious daughter and the scary part of the journey that we had been heading towards was about to begin. Would I get to hold her in my arms, pink and warm, hear her cry and feel her warm body against mine? Would she survive?

Our arrival at the event resulted in the most memorable introduction ever. *"Hello, this is my wife. She's in labour, but don't worry, she's just going to sit over there and get on with it!"*

I still chuckle over this one now, and my husband has never lived it down! He did also add that I was a midwife and that as long as I was calm, he was calm. Once I started getting worried, he would start getting worried!

I waited in the crew catering room while my husband set up the event. He popped in a few times to check that I was okay. The contractions were still fairly infrequent and mild but were starting to get stronger. At midday, I told my husband that I was ready to go. His dad had now been briefed and was ready to take over running the event. It was an hour's drive down the motorway to the hospital where Jessica would be born. It wasn't our local hospital but the one I had trained at as a student midwife. We had chosen to go there as it was next door to a hospital with specialist children's cardiac facilities. I knew that it was still early on labour-wise though, so we stopped en-route for lunch at the motorway services.

We arrived at the hospital at around 2.00pm. The midwife that met us was one I'd worked with as a student. It felt very strange to be on the other side! I was examined and was 1cm dilated. As I'd suspected, it was still early days and so I was transferred to the antenatal ward to wait for my labour to progress.

As the afternoon moved towards evening, my contractions became stronger. I could also feel pressure in my lower back which became harder and harder to bear. By 8.00pm I was struggling to breathe through the contractions. I needed something more.

The midwife came and examined me. I was 2cm. I burst into tears. I knew that the contractions were still too spaced out for me to be far along but the pressure in my back was excruciating. The midwife gave me gas and air. I tried to breathe on it but I didn't like the way it made me feel. I felt drunk, as though I was observing the situation from far away. The contractions felt exactly the same as they had felt before so I started breathing on the gas and air, but I felt slightly paralysed and unable to voice how I was feeling. I didn't like it at all.

After a while I was transferred to the labour ward. The pressure in my back was now unbearable and I was starting to get uncontrollable urges to push. I wanted an epidural. I was examined again – 5cm. Too soon to be pushing, but no matter how hard I tried, I couldn't stop myself pushing. The anaesthetist arrived to put the epidural in. Thankfully the epidural started taking effect quite quickly. I was still aware of the contractions, was still aware of my body spontaneously pushing, but it was all quite manageable now.

It was now midnight. My husband settled down in a reclining chair and fell asleep. I was encouraged to sleep too but I was too tuned into the noises of the CTG (heart-rate) monitor. Every time Jessica's heart rate dropped slightly, my eyes flew open. Thankfully, once I was turned on to my side, her heart rate picked back up again.

After a few hours, I was examined again. I was still 5cm and so the midwife started me on a syntocinon drip. The next time I was examined, I was 9cm. I had requested for Jessica to be baptised as soon as possible after birth due to her poor prognosis and the hospital chaplain was called ready for this. I started to feel anxious again at the thought of what might happen when Jessica was born.

By 6.00am, I was ready to push and the midwives woke my husband up so he could support me. I tried hard to push through each contraction, but as time went on, it seemed that Jessica was no closer to being born. The team were concerned that I shouldn't push for too long because of Jessica's heart condition and so they decided that she would need some help from forceps to be born.

The room was suddenly full of people – paediatricians, obstetricians, midwives. As Jessica was born she was placed on my tummy – pink, warm and crying. I burst into tears and sobbed uncontrollably.

She was here, she was pink, she was crying! She was alive and she was utterly beautiful. After the briefest and most beautiful cuddle, Jessica was taken over to the resuscitaire in the corner of the room where she was checked over and baptised. Once she was checked over, she was wrapped in the towel and I got to have another cuddle for a few minutes before she was taken to the neonatal unit.

We had another cuddle later that day in the neonatal unit before Jessica was transferred to the general hospital for open-heart surgery at just eight hours old. She spent four weeks in hospital recovering before we finally got to take her home. Her birth was much more medicalised than I would have hoped for, but the midwives and doctors who cared for me were wonderful. That moment, when Jessica was born and I heard her cry, was one of the most joyful moments of my whole life.

Sophie's Birth

My second pregnancy was a very different experience! We had extra scans to check the baby's heart, but thankfully all seemed to be well. We had found out Jessica's gender at twenty weeks because of her heart condition, but this time around we chose to wait until our baby was born to find out. Two of my independent midwife friends agreed to be my midwives. We hired a heated birth pool which was set up ready in our dining room. We had a little hiccup when we first filled it due to a faulty part, which meant we almost flooded our dining room but thankfully a replacement part was sent out quickly and the pool was set up successfully the second time. These pools are no longer recommended as they carry an increased risk for Legionnaire's disease, but we didn't know that at the time!

Although I had gone into labour at thirty-eight weeks with Jessica, this baby seemed to be much comfier inside the big mamma house. My due date came and went. A few days later, as the clocks went back after British Summertime, my labour started. It was an hour or so after the first contraction that I realised that this was the real thing and not another bout of Braxton Hicks contractions (as I'd been having over the previous few weeks). I woke my husband up to help me put on the TENS machine. A few contractions later, we decided it was time to phone the midwives. My husband also phoned my mum and my twin sister so that they could head over to be with us and to look after Jessica who was fast asleep in her cot.

By the time my first midwife arrived, I was in the pool downstairs. The water was warm and soothing and whilst the contractions felt intense, I could focus and breathe through them. My husband had put my relaxing birth music on and was kneeling by the side of the pool, holding my hands during the contractions and giving me hugs in between.

My mum and twin sister arrived a little while later. Jessica woke up shortly after their arrival so Mum went upstairs to see to her and then brought her downstairs a little while later. She wasn't at all bothered by Mummy being in labour – she came over to me saying "*Mummy*" and gave me a big kiss. Then she went into the lounge with Nanny where she could play with her toys. Every so often Jessica would come to the gate between the lounge and dining room and look at me and say "*Mummy!*" and then go back and play. She wasn't fazed by it at all.

As the contractions got stronger and more frequent, I felt myself retreating further inward, really needing to concentrate on getting through them. My husband continued to be there for me to cuddle and hold his hands as I needed. My twin occasionally offered a few words of reassurance but mostly everyone was just there, being quietly supportive which was exactly what I needed them to be doing.

As it started to get light outside, I was beginning to feel scared and overwhelmed, feeling like I couldn't do it. My midwives reassured me that I was doing well. The contractions were starting to space out a little though. My midwives wondered if I was distracted by Jessica being nearby and suggested that my mum take her upstairs for a while. I hoped that this was a good sign that everyone thought baby's arrival might be imminent!

I was beginning to feel much more '*pushy*' now and the sensation was overwhelming me, frightening me. I didn't want to do this anymore. I was scared of tearing, scared of something going wrong. I wanted it all to stop and go away for a bit, to give me a breather, but I knew that if it stopped, I would never want it to start again!

The pushing stage felt so long. I had thought second time around the pushing stage would be quick but this seemed so slow – taking three steps forward and two back every time. And then I heard my midwives telling me "*little pushes now.*"

Nearly there. I felt a little pop and knew baby's head was out. One more contraction, another big push and relief as I felt my baby's body emerge from me into the water.

Somebody was telling me to lift my baby out of the water and then suddenly there were two beautiful dark eyes blinking up at me. Joy flooded over me as I looked at this precious little bundle in my arms. I looked down and saw we had another girl, our little Sophie.

She wasn't crying yet though. I blew in her face and rubbed her little arms to encourage her to take that big first breath. And then she screwed up her little face and gave a big cry, much to my relief. I couldn't move her very much, it was all I could do just to keep her little face above the water as her cord felt quite short.

Mum brought Jessica downstairs. "*Baby!*" Jessica exclaimed when she saw Sophie. She was fascinated as she stood on the step next to the pool with Daddy holding her, looking down at her new sister and giving me a big kiss.

The midwives clamped Sophie's cord and my husband cut it. I had decided to wait for the placenta to come out naturally. After an hour though, it still hadn't emerged and I was finding the sensation of having it still inside quite uncomfortable so opted for the injection to help deliver it.

After a nice warm bath, it was lovely to be able to get into my own bed and snuggle with my new baby. I did enjoy my '*babymoon*', pretty much staying in bed for a week (on my midwives' advice), whilst my husband looked after us all. It was wonderful to feel cocooned in my home for that first week. It was such a different experience to Jessica's birth, but no more or less special because of it.

Louise George's Labour Tips:

- If all seems well, try and stay at home for as long as possible, especially if it is your first baby.

- Try and stay as relaxed and calm as possible. Focusing on breathing through the contractions and counting through the breath really helped me. Having a warm bath can also help.

- If you feel like you need pain relief, don't be afraid to ask for it.

- Try and go with the flow. Every labour is different and babies don't read birth plans!

- Have confidence in yourself and focus on the thought of having your baby in your arms. Each contraction is one contraction nearer to that point.

Louise George's Biography

Louise is a mum to two little girls. Her eldest daughter was born with hypoplastic left heart syndrome and her youngest is heart-healthy. She blogs about parenthood and life as a '*heart*' family over at http://littleheartsbiglove.co.uk and is passionate about raising awareness of congenital heart defects.

By Becky O'Haire, Cuddle Fairy Blog

My Story

Hi, I'm Becky, creator and author of CuddleFairy.com. I live in the West of Ireland but I am originally from New York. I have three kiddies who are now 10, 7 and 4. All three of them were born in Ireland.

I'm excited to share my birth stories with you today! I think the best thing that women can do is to tell their birth stories and talk about how they felt after giving birth too – there is so much that just isn't spoken about. The reality of giving birth and the feelings that go along with it are immense. It's a huge thing for your body to do, just think about it!

I say that now... but ten years ago, I gave no thought to my first pregnancy. I was twenty-seven and carried on in life as normal, until I started having heart palpitations in the third trimester. I was told that was normal in pregnancy until one day, in the doctor's office, I had a resting heartbeat of 144bpm. I was sent straight to the hospital and was put on a beta blocker.

I took the meds and I followed along with the rest of my pregnancy without looking into the medication, I didn't google it. It's crazy to say this now, but this was pre-smart phones. I used to go to an internet café to send emails!! Yikes, how the times have changed, now I google everything via my phone!

Anyway, my due date arrived and I was given a sweep that day. I felt awful afterwards and swore I'd never have a sweep pre-labour again. That evening I started having regular pains. By 2.00am they were every five minutes so we headed to the hospital.

The midwife examined me and I was 1 cm. ONE. I couldn't believe that was all, but they said I was in labour so they kept me in. I walked around the hospital grounds all day long. The pain really kicked off that afternoon and I was struggling to walk anymore or hold any conversation with the other women in the ward. But oddly enough, I never asked for pain meds. It's like I was in a fog.

The nurses were super busy and didn't check me again until 4.00pm that afternoon when I was 2cm. It felt like all of the walking was for nothing, because nothing was happening, yet the pain was coming.

They put a trace on my belly and found out that our baby was distressed. Basically, he wasn't enjoying all of the contractions without any progression. I was brought into a labour room where they broke my waters. It was extremely painful and I had no pain medicine which I also vowed I'd never let happen again.

Once the waters broke the contractions took off at top speed. They were coming every twenty seconds and I just couldn't cope. The pain was immense and I decided to have an epidural, something I wasn't intending to have. But I didn't know how long labour would continue on for since I was only 2cm and the pain was so bad. So, I decided to take the epidural. Being honest, if someone offered to hit me over the head with a frying pan I would have taken that too!

The epidural was glorious, after four more hours of labour and half an hour of pushing, our gorgeous son was born weighing 9lbs 4oz. It was an unassisted natural birth, as my following two births also were.

As you can probably guess, with such a big first baby, I had a lot of stitches – the doctor pulled up a chair and was there stitching for a loooong time.

The next morning, our son turned purple and was rushed to special care. His blood sugar had crashed. I discovered later, that low blood sugar for the baby is a side effect of the beta blockers I was taking. I was really upset that no one was looking out for this or expecting it!

I went into a state of depression. I didn't realize it at the time but I started to cry that day and didn't stop for about two weeks. I cried over everything. I felt inadequate, I worried he wasn't getting enough milk as I was breastfeeding. Everything was a worry and I was so delirious from not sleeping for three nights and being in labour for so long that I just couldn't think straight.

Thank goodness, our son was only in special care for a few days. The nurses in there were amazing and they were the ones who taught me how to breastfeed properly. After a few weeks of feeling blue at home, things became bright for me again.

It took about nine months before I stopped being sore when I sat down. I started to think it'd be like that forever but it wasn't. It's important to realize your body has gone through something big and you have to give yourself plenty of time to recover. And give yourself a break too, don't be critical or hard on how you feel.

Fast forward two years and five months and I was back at the hospital ready to give birth to our second son. I went in there ready to not allow certain things to happen again – I had learned some lessons with our first son. I was on beta blockers again and had the entire hospital told about it and to watch our baby's blood sugar.

This time around my waters broke themselves around 5.00am. I walked around the hospital all day again – it was quite familiar. That night the pains kicked off. Again, I didn't think to ask for pain killers. The fog of labour pains had descended upon me again. I just asked if I could ring my husband to come back. Yes, they had made my husband go home at 9.00pm.

I remember so clearly calling my husband at 2.00am. He was there at 2.30am and our son was born at 3.30am. There was no time for an epidural so I just ploughed ahead. I didn't manage the pain that well, it felt out of my control, but luckily it went so quickly and it was all over soon.

Our second son flew out with a few pushes at 8lbs 15oz. There were only a few stitches and an easy recovery. Breastfeeding was easier the second time around. Our son's blood sugar didn't crash because we were careful and monitored his feeds and his sugar levels. The whole experience was much more positive and I didn't have any blues after his birth. I think it was a much more positive experience because I had learned so much the first time around.

Fast forward three years and five months later and I was back in maternity yet again with baby number three, our precious little girl. I was older and wiser this time around. Before her pregnancy, I had a round of acupuncture. During her pregnancy, I rested as my GP advised me to do. These two things enabled me to stay off the beta blockers, which was a big relief, as there wasn't concerns over her blood sugar levels.

During her labour I meditated, saying the same few lines over and over to myself. I found that helped me so much. I used the gas and air which I enjoyed that time. With the boys' labours I took a few puffs from the gas and air, but felt it was making me light headed. The third time around, I learned to keep puffing and it gets better!

I was in labour on February 13th. Our daughter was born at 11.57pm that evening. I remember when she was born asking what time it was because I wasn't sure if she was going to be a Valentine's Day baby or not! She decided to have her own day instead.

Our daughter weighted 9lbs 15oz. There was a lot of pushing involved which I didn't think would happen being the third child, but she was a full pound heavier than her big brother. Miraculously I didn't need any stitches! The midwife who delivered our daughter was so supportive and gave me space. My waters didn't break until 10cm and I was pushing. I think having the waters in tact made the labour less painful than the boys where my water was broken. Out of the three deliveries, hers was the calmest for me.

My three birth stories, for me, are about the learning and growing I did as an individual and as a mother. The most important things are that all three of my kids were healthy. Nothing else really matters at the end of the day. For any future parents reading this, I hope you are kind to yourself. Take it easy, be your own advocate and best of luck to you on your journey ahead!

Pregnancy & Labour Tips:

* Rest and be kind to yourself during your pregnancy.

* Research any medicines you are given and make sure all doctors and nurses are aware of what you are taking and any possible side effects.

* Do your own research on having a sweep done on your due date to see if it's right for you.

* Be your own advocate and ask for help, ask for medicine, ask to be checked.

* Allow yourself to take medicines if you need them during labour.

* Be flexible with your birth plan.

* Walking during labour was helpful in all three of my births.

* Try to keep your labour partner in the hospital if you can. If not, be sure to call them asap if pains kick off.

* Having a meditation or a few lines to say over and over was very helpful to me.

Becky O'Haire's Biography

Becky is the author and creator at Cuddle Fairy (www.cuddlefairy.com), a parenting and lifestyle blog that focuses on positivity. Becky writes about family travels, parenting, shares recipes and much more. Cuddle Fairy's motto is: there's positivity around every corner. Really and truly your mindset is everything. Cuddle Fairy looks to the positive. You can find Becky on her blog and Cuddle Fairy's social media networks:

Facebook – (https://www.facebook.com/cuddlefairy)

Twitter - (https://twitter.com/CuddleFairy) and

YouTube - (https://www.youtube.com/c/CuddleFairy1).

Reneé Davis – Wife, Mama, Author, Blogger

http://mummytries.com

When I gave birth for the third time, it was as straight forward as childbirth gets. I had my first strong contraction at around 12.00pm, one day after my due date. My husband and I arrived at the birthing centre attached to our local hospital just before 4.00pm. I was already 5cm dilated and Freddy was born within three hours. I pushed him out in less than half an hour without the need for drugs or medical attention afterwards.

I gave birth for the second time two years and four days previous to that. Giving birth to Clara wasn't as fast and I needed the help of gas and pethidine for the pain. I discovered that I was holding onto trauma from the first time around and I would push her out a little bit, get scared and then suck her back in. This went on for an hour and a half, but I managed to push her out and felt incredibly proud of myself for doing so.

My first experience was another story entirely...

We'd planned a home birth for Polly, but after a five-day early labour, and spending twelve hours in established labour, it became apparent that things were not going to pan out the way I hoped they would. My baby was stuck and we needed a blue light to the hospital.

Fortunately, I had a fantastically experienced community midwife with me throughout and never once felt scared. It was through her insistence that I received an epidural when I arrived at the hospital (even though I was 9cm dilated). The respite gave me the chance to rest while I was put onto a syntocinon drip, to bring on the contractions.

I pushed for almost two hours and Polly was delivered with forceps. I haemorrhaged quite badly afterwards and was stitched from vagina to anus. It was a shock to discover my first baby was almost 9lb, as everyone had predicted a 6lb baby for a small lady like me (I'm a mere 5'2"). She was also back to back, which explained why she got so stuck.

Had the midwife not made the call to get to hospital when she did, who knows how things would have worked out for us both. I'll be eternally grateful for being looked after as well as I was.

Reneé Davis' Biography

Wife and mum of three, Reneé Davis blogs at 'Mummy Tries', about the non-sugar-coated ups and downs of family life. Among other things, Reneé is a home educator, autism mama, mental health advocate and real food enthusiast. As the survivor of a dysfunctional childhood, she has undergone quite a journey to ensure that her children have a better start to life than the one she had.

Her memoir/self-help book, 'Become the Best You' has lots of practical advice to help others break cycles of negativity and dysfunction. Reneé is currently working on her first novel, a roller coaster ride through motherhood and mental health, called '*Picking up the Pieces*'.

Reneé Davis
Wife, mama, author, blogger
http://mummytries.com
http://amzn.to/1N2ZnMn
http://www.huffingtonpost.co.uk/author/renee-davis

Knife to Skin. My Birth Story by Catherine Balavage

So, now we get to my birth story. It was written long after the other contributors because I kept putting it off. When I got pregnant I was going to write a book on pregnancy, but then my pregnancy was so awful and so unlike most women's pregnancies that I decided not to. I did not want to scare women by writing about my terrible pregnancy. I felt much the same about the labour. My labour was very unique. Over eighty hours of hell followed by an emergency C-section. There was a catalogue of errors from the hospital, along with a lot of bullying. The best part of the actual birth was getting gutted, like a shark that had ate a small human being. Of course, the moment my son was put on my chest it was all worth it. My husband says he will never forget the look on my face. It was, without a doubt, the best moment of my life. I cried tears of pure joy and I do not care how corny that sounds.

My son's birth started on a Sunday evening. The contractions started. I told my husband who was excited. He went to build the cot. I thought my baby would be born soon. How naive I was. In-between contractions I text my parents to say that I was in labour. They started their long journey down from Scotland soon after. I hoped they would arrive in time for the birth. I called the hospital who told me to take some paracetamol and go for a bath.

I went to bed that night having semi-regular contractions. I did not get any sleep. I was full of nerves. Both excited and scared. The next day I was in labour all day. My contractions were regular. The hospital gave the same advice: stay home. On the Tuesday things were getting tough. After two sleepless nights and countless contractions I was finding it hard. The pain seemed to be getting worse and the contractions were still regular, every few minutes.

I called the hospital who just gave me the same advice. I went to the bathroom and had a shower. When the mucus plug came away, I was so excited. I initially thought my waters had broken when this happened, but not so lucky. Again, I called the hospital. The woman who answered the phone told me to come in and they would see me, with a weary and slightly annoyed tone to her voice. They made me feel like I was wasting their time. They had no compassion for the fact I was a first-time mother in labour.

We went to the hospital and I thought that this might finally be it. It turns out I was only 2cm dilated. There was one nice midwife who was considerate. She told me my waters had broken (they had not) and offered to do a membrane sweep. I was not sure what that was but I agreed. I was then sent home so I would not use up *'valuable NHS resources.'* I guess it did not matter that I was a tax payer.

The next day everything ramped up again. After another sleepless night I was struggling. My husband called the hospital, I called the hospital and eventually, by the evening, they allowed me to return. I was given some pethidine to help my sleep but they forgot to give me the anti-nausea pill that went with it. I spent the rest of my labour throwing up and feeling dizzy. I was unable to even drink without throwing up. On Wednesday evening my midwife came in with a face of thunder. She yelled and screamed at me, telling me I should be at home and I was wasting NHS resources. She said she would be splitting the room as another patient was coming in. While she was screaming my waters started breaking. This did not stop her. She continued to bully me and scream, while giving me evil looks. *'You should be at home'* she said, while my waters gushed out.

Later I will read in my birth notes that the midwife was told to split the room and that *'Catherine understands'* and it filled me with rage. My birth records read like a work of fiction. I mention this to other mothers, including some who had their babies in the same hospital, and they agree. I take her disgusting tirade with politeness and a smile. My mother looks on, helpless and upset. Neither of us complain as we are too scared of the consequences. The bully and an eye-rolling accomplice split the room in two and change my bed sheets after my waters broke all over them. A small revenge it seems. After they leave I dig deep for any positivity and there it is: I was told a baby has to born within twenty-four hours of a women's water breaking, otherwise there is an increased risk of infection. I allow myself a small smile. Just one more day.

My contractions are still regular and intense. I had been timing them the entire time. In pencil and paper there it is: two-three minutes apart. Increasing in pain and intensity. I feel an intense pain crawl up my back. I call the midwife. The only one who is nice and seems to care at all comes in. I tell her the pain is ramping up and I don't know what is happening. She says I can only have one more dose of pethidine. I don't want any more but the pain is intense and I agree. A little while afterwards I hear the same bully midwife from the water-breaking scenario say directly outside my room, *'Jeez, how much more pethidine is that baby going to have.'*

I want to punch her, but I don't have the energy. I have been in labour for days and have had no sleep. After a while, I ask to talk to a midwife about progress and options. She says if I have not given birth by 8.00am the following day they will induce me. At last I have a finish line. It is what I needed more than anything: knowing that this will end. I put my iPod on and listen to my music, while my poor husband, who has never left my side for a moment, spends another night trying to sleep in an uncomfortable chair. I count down the hours until 8.00am. Ten hours later it happens. It was possibly the longest ten hours of my life. I press on the button to call the midwife and I do not let go. I am determined to keep them at their word.

It takes a little while but a midwife does come. She is pretty and blonde and has a kind face. She is the start of proper treatment. She is everything a midwife actually should be. She will stay with me, even hours later. She tells me that they are changing the staff over and she had heard I had been having a hard time. After they change the staff and exchange notes she will be back. I smile. Not long after she comes in and puts a fetal monitor across my stomach. She then leaves to do something. As I lie there I hear the baby's heartbeat, and then I don't. It keeps dropping. At first, I am too scared to acknowledge it, but then I mention it to my husband. *'Press the button'* he says. I do and I do not let go.

It is at this point everything changes. The NHS is no longer useless. But, of course, that is the NHS. Good in a crisis and so, so otherwise. The same midwife comes in. My husband is standing. I can see that underneath the calmness he is projecting for my benefit that there is panic in his eyes. I am doing the same thing. Staying calm for my husband and my son. Keeping the terror down. We tell the midwife about the heart monitor. She doesn't hide her panic. She gets someone else. I am transferred to the labour ward while being constantly monitored. I had been drinking Lucozade non-stop as one of the midwives told me it would help. The midwives now tell me it is full of caffeine and sugar and is *'the worst'*. I also spent hours bouncing up and down on a birthing ball and walking around. It is fair to say that none of this advice worked.

When we finally get to the labour ward they ask if I want gas and air. I say I am worried it will make me dizzy. *'Everything we have causes nausea unfortunately'* they tell me. Anyway. I have been in labour for days. I request an epidural. The moment I get it, it is one of the best moments of my life. It WORKS. Nothing else I had - pethidine, paracetamol (as if!) - worked. I ask how much longer it takes once a woman gets to the labour ward. *'About twelves hours'* they tell me. I almost give up hope. Well, until I got the epidural. After that it was hard to care. They finally begin to induce me and then things happen quickly. Baby does not like it and gets further in distress. The surgeon comes, the anaesthetist comes. Everything is go now. Everything is serious. I sign the forms and am whisked off to theatre. As I head through the doors I feel like a failure. I could not give birth to my own baby. My body had failed me. My worst fear had been a C-section and now here I was: about to be gutted like a shark that had swallowed a mini surfer. I had walked past the theatre trying to move the labour along, so happy I was not having surgery. Ha, ha to me. But now it seems to happen quickly. I am terrified of course. But then I see his head. Then he is bundled out and wrapped in a blanket and given to me. This is the best moment. This is everything. This is my son. Every moment, every second, was worth it. I look at him and I cannot believe he is real.

My labour was terrible so I do not want you to read this and think it is going to happen to you. I do not know any other women this has happened to. From the Thursday morning, when the new midwife came everything was different. I was given the best care and treated with respect. The surgeon who was female was great and so was the team in general. The truth was, I was unlucky. It took me a year to work up the courage to have a birth review and it was awful. The first thing the woman said to me was *'you took a lot of drugs, didn't you?'* She also said the labour did not count as I spent too long in early labour. There was no apology for how they treated me or their catalogue of errors. Just defensiveness and blame. It was awful and left me angry. A while later I paid to get a copy of my birth records: in my opinion they read like a work of fiction. The truth there does not belong to me. It is only when I see another consultant at a different hospital during my second pregnancy - an amazing woman - that she tells me that my son was back-to-back and that makes labour more difficult and painful. She went through the notes with me and explained things. It made such a difference.

My son is two now. I am thankful that I did not get Post Traumatic Stress Disorder (PTSD) or Post Natal Depression (PND) from the birth. I had a bad labour but I have a wonderful son. I have no regrets.

Just Breathe. My Second Birth Story

When you have a previous caesarean section, you have a choice of a planned caesarean section, or a VBAC (vaginal birth after previous caesarean section), I had many appointments with the consultant and we had agreed that if I had not given birth by the 16th of October, they would check my cervix and give me a sweep. Then I would have a planned caesarean section on the 17th of October. My due date was the 7th of October. I had to be heavily monitored as there was a small risk - about one in two hundred - that the scar on my uterus would rupture. On Thursday the 28th of September they checked my cervix and my cervix was *'sky high'*. They did not expect labour to be anytime soon. Two days later I went into labour. Four days later, our daughter was born.

My second labour started in Waitrose. I had period-like cramps all day and when I got my first contraction I thought it was Braxton hicks. We had lunch in the cafe and then went to the park. Later on, we watched a movie together as a family. I was dead on thirty-nine weeks. My son was forty-one plus three, so I was not expecting our daughter to come early. I had been eating dates from thirty-seven weeks onwards, as many people had recommended them, saying that they softened the cervix and made labour shorter. I had also been drinking raspberry leaf tea, until I read in a few articles that you should not drink it if you have had a previous caesarean section, or are having another one. I asked my consultant about it, but she had never heard of it. I stopped anyway to be safe.

I had also stayed very active. Walking as much as possible even though the baby felt very uncomfortable and heavy towards the end. I believe the combination of the dates, staying fit, and doing breathing during my contractions made the difference in my second labour. I was still unsure whether I was in labour when we went to bed that night. I had called the hospital and they said it was either Braxton hicks, or the start of labour. I was to keep them informed. In the early hours of Sunday there was no more denying it. I was in labour and having contractions. We got the toddler and put him in the pram and we all went to the hospital. We could not find a taxi so we had to take the night bus. When I got there, they hooked me up to the monitor and confirmed that I was in labour. I was sent home and told to come back when the contractions were closer together. I called my parents who started their journey from Scotland to look after the toddler. I spent Saturday morning in the bath trying to alleviate the pain, reading a book, while the rest of the family slept. I also took paracetamol.

It was not until Saturday afternoon that contractions got stronger and I went back to the hospital. I was 2cm, the baby's head was down and my cervix was thin. All good signs. I felt a bit more positive and hoped that this labour would be quick. The contractions got more and more intense as the day got on. My parents arrived about noon which made things easier. I had to take the night bus twice while in labour and now my dad could drive me and they could look after our son. Thanks mum and dad! '*I think we will see you tonight*' the midwife had said. She was not wrong. We went home and in the end, went to bed. Not long after we went to bed my waters broke and we went back to the hospital. The contractions were getting stronger and more frequent. It was a busy night in the hospital. They were still dealing with the aftermath of the September baby boom; more babies are born in that month than any other. People get amorous during Christmas and New Year apparently.

The night our daughter was born, another thirteen babies were born. But in the waiting room I knew something was happening. I felt an urge to push. I told my husband to get the midwife and they came and helped me to a room. They checked me by feeling my stomach and said I was getting the urge to push as the baby was transversal and slightly back-to-back. This made my heart sink. My son had been in the same position and I had been told that was partly why his birth had gone so badly. I tried to stay as relaxed as possible and breathe through the contractions. With my first birth, I was in the first stage for five days and the hospital were not helpful. I did not know, nor was told how, to deal with the contractions. The midwives now, however, kept saying how well I was doing. The entire staff were amazing and supportive during my entire labour. I could not have had a better midwife and the doctor was also amazing. They checked and I was 4cm. They asked if I wanted any gas and air. I tried some, but found it distracting rather than helpful. I found it easier to cope with the contractions by breathing through them. I turned down the other pain relief. In my opinion the only thing that works is the epidural and I was too scared it would slow down the birth.

By now I had been in labour for a while and the contractions felt very intense and strong. I had hit the wall. I knew I could be in labour for hours and decided that I could not take anymore. With the midwife's encouragement I decided to have an epidural. My heart sank however, when they said the anaesthetist had just gone into theatre. I figured it was probably for a caesarean section and they generally take forty-five minutes. It would be an hour until I got an epidural. I decided to suck it up and deal with it. All pain is temporary I told myself, this too shall pass I also told myself. Lastly, I kept reminding myself that childbirth is a privilege. Many women want a child and do not get one.

Then something amazing happened, even though it did not feel like it at the time. I kept pushing even when I tried not to. The midwife checked me again. I was 8cm. In no time at all I was on my back being told to push. It was intense and painful but I pushed and at 3.35am our daughter was born. I had to have an episiotomy to help the baby come out quicker. I also made the mistake of pushing when I was not having a contraction because I was worried that the baby was not coming fast enough, which think made the situation worse. That is how you tear. Not fun. Tip: only push when you are having a contraction or when the midwife tells you. The next thing I knew I was told the head was out, which stung a little but was not that bad. For one moment I worried as there was no crying but I just waited for the next contraction to push some more. Then I did and there she was: our daughter. They put her on top of me and I can honestly say that the moments where I met my children for the first time are the greatest of my life. There is no other feeling like it. They put her on top of me and I fell completely in love. She was there and yet I could not believe it. It was surreal. We felt even luckier as I had a heavy bleed early in the pregnancy, and we were told there was a thirty to forty per cent chance she had died. We had to wait until the next day to get a scan and see if she was still alive. Then she was in our arms and our dreams came true again.

Luckily the placenta came out fairly easily. I only had to push twice and the midwife pulled some of it out. My husband also cut the cord. My husband had been so supportive and wonderful during the entire process, telling me to breathe and push. The funniest part of the birth was him telling me to breathe and me yelling '*no!*' at him. He told me later I even started saying no to the midwife. He was amazing the entire time. Now we were a family of four and so happy. The amazing midwife, who I will always be eternally grateful to, then got us some tea and some bread and jam, to give us time together as a family. She then came back and sewed up my nether regions. It was painful and took about forty-five minutes, but I was so tired I actually fell asleep a few times while she was doing it. My second birth was the VBAC I wanted and I felt happy and proud, but I also felt lucky. Because sometimes a good birth is merely that. But I did do everything I could to tip the odds in my favour. So, read on for my tips.

- Find out how to breathe through the contractions. There are Hypnobirthing tips from Paola Bagnall below. It made a huge difference to my labour. Do not hold your breath or tense. Try and stay as relaxed and calm as possible. Easier said than done, but it does make a difference.

- Eat dates. I have no idea if they did work but I do not think it was a coincidence that I ate at least six a day from thirty-seven weeks and my labour was much shorter and easier.

- Get and stay, as fit as possible. It has been proven that exercising and staying fit during pregnancy means a shorter labour. Pregnancy and labour are hard on the body so staying fit and healthy is important.

- Make sure you relax as much as possible. Preserve your energy for when you will need it.

- Stay hydrated and eat carbs.

- Try to not panic. Keep as calm as possible.

- Remember that all pain is temporary. You will soon meet your baby and every moment will be worth it. Stay positive. You can do this.

- Trust your body.

- If you need drugs then ask for them. If you cannot take the pain then tell the midwife. There is no shame in it. Childbirth hurts. Do what is right for you. If the birth does not go the way you wanted it to, do not beat yourself up about it. Nothing was your fault. You have done an amazing thing. Feel proud of yourself and rest as much as possible.

- If you had to have an episiotomy then take pain killers. Pour a jug of warm water over yourself when you pee to stop the stinging, and bath your lower regions in tea tree oil for ten to fifteen minutes a day. Remember to shower and keep the area clean so you do not get an infection. Another good tip is to clench your bottom when sitting down or getting up. Try and do your pelvic floor exercises as soon as possible. It helps blood flow to the area and speeds up healing.

Milli Hill of The Positive Birth Movement

There aren't many mysteries left in life, but predicting when a baby is going to turn up still seems to be one of them. I can still remember the day when, pregnant with my third baby, I was one-day shy of forty-two weeks pregnant. At this point, I was liable to burst into hysterical laughter or tears without warning and was wider sideways than I was tall. It seemed like I would be pregnant forever.

That night, just before I set off on the long journey on my hands and knees to bed, I remembered that the following morning was the first day back at school for my five-year-old daughter. *"I think I'd rather have a baby than get up and make a packed lunch"*, I thought to myself. And that is precisely what happened.

It didn't start the way I expected, with the slow build-up of tightening I'd had before. Instead, a soap opera beginning: ten minutes after getting into bed, a mild contraction, then a pop, then a flood of waters. Myself and my partner hid in the bathroom, dealing with the torrent of giggling, whispering, and trying not to wake the other two children.

I cried a bit too. I felt daunted by the task that lay ahead and scared by this curve ball beginning that I hadn't expected. What else would surprise me in this labour? I think I'm like most modern women – I don't like surprises. I'd rather be in control. Labour doesn't allow this. It's all about letting go. So, I breathed out, and I cried.

Later, we tried to return to bed, but I knew in my heart that this was pointless and that I needed to get up and face the music. I texted our midwife and by 3.00am she was with us, full of reassurance as we all drank tea on the sofa. She told me that labouring women had to go to the stars to bring back the soul of their baby, and sent me and my partner off for a dip in the birth pool while she knitted a baby hat in another room. It sounds idyllic, but really, this is exactly what happened!

In a back room of our house, we had a beautiful heated pool ready and waiting, and we floated for an hour or two in the candlelight, listening to my favourite Joni Mitchell albums. Her voice seemed to carry me up and away from the pain of contractions, as my partner kept me feeling loved and grounded in between.

Later on, the intensity started to build and things got tough. Sometimes I rode the wave and sometimes I thought I would drown in it. I gripped tight to my man, who knelt outside the pool now, and wished it would all just end. At times I thought I could not go on, and at times I felt like a warrior, never stronger. Towards the end, there were more polar opposites: the feeling that I would die or split in two…and the blissful sensation of my baby turning, wriggling, and swimming out of me into the waters of the pool.

And then it was done and he was in my arms, meeting my gaze with bright eyes, and there was only one feeling: exhilaration.

Women like me who have births like this are often described as *'lucky'*. A friend who heard my story last week remarked, *"wow, birth is obviously just 'your thing', you were made to do it!"*. Of course, it's true that sometimes we can be unlucky in birth – when mother nature deals us wild cards that mean medical intervention is necessary. So, in this sense, I was lucky.

But this aside, I can assure you that there is nothing special about me, and that the majority of women can be lucky and experience the roller coaster ride of exhilarating birth, just as I did. We are all made of roughly the same stuff, and, with some good planning and preparation, we can all cry, laugh, struggle and triumph through the agony and ecstasy of childbirth. We can all go to the stars and bring back our baby's souls, as women have for millennia. Because birth is not just '*my thing*' – with luck on our side, we were all '*made to do it*'.

http://www.positivebirthmovement.org

The Positive Birth movement is an amazing movement to take the fear out of childbirth and support women. They have 250 groups in the UK and over 200 in the rest of the world. It is a global network of free to attend antenatal groups which are linked up by social media. They bring pregnant women together to share stories, expertise and positivity about childbirth. They aim to take away the negativity and fear surrounding modern childbirth, and help change things for the better. Join them and also buy Milli's book which I have read and love: Positive Birth Book.https://www.amazon.co.uk/d/Books/Positive-Birth-New-Approach-Pregnancy-Early-Weeks/1780664303/

I hope you enjoyed the stories and tips contained in this book. Please feel free to share your own birth stories and send any comments to: frostmagazine@gmail.com.
If you would like your birth story published in a future book or in Frost Magazine, then please add '*for publication*' in your email. Thank you and good luck!

Top Ten tips on How to Use Self-Hypnosis for Birth Hypnobirthing
By Paola Bagnall

Hypnobirthing is simply a generic term that means the use of hypnosis for birth. There are several different forms of hypnobirthing, which all work towards helping the mum have a natural birth.

We are all in hypnosis, without knowing it, about 60% of the day, so this is something that comes naturally to us all. It occurs just before you fall asleep and just as you awaken. Other examples include losing track of time when reading a good book, when watching something interesting on television, or when you do anything you enjoy doing. Have you ever driven from A to B, arrived at your destination and not remembered how you drove there? If so, you were in the daydreaming state of natural hypnosis.

In essence, hypnosis is simply a state of heightened relaxation and altered awareness. In hypnosis you are awake, aware of what is going on around you and you are in control. It is all to do with the mind-body connection.

Hypnobirthing is based on the work of Dr Grantly Dick-Read, an English Physician whose principles provided the foundations of the National Childbirth Trust (NCT). He is famously quoted as saying; "*In no other animal species is the process of birth apparently associated with any suffering, pain or agony, except where pathology exists or in an unnatural state, such as captivity.*" He went on to conclude that fear and tension was responsible for 95% of labour pain, which could be eliminated through relaxation techniques.

Hypnobirthing is the intended use of natural hypnosis to allow you to tap into your inner resources, which we all have in our unconscious minds, to create feelings of well-being. When you are relaxed you cannot feel fear and so birth becomes a more enjoyable process, a magical experience which the female body is beautifully designed to achieve biologically.

Hypnobirthing helps you to: -

- Put things into their true perspective;
- Relax, stay calm and in control - in a calm, relaxed state your muscles and skin can stretch easily and naturally in a pain-free way;
- Stay focused on the process that your body is going through and be in tune with what your body and your intuition are telling you;
- Be healthy and sleep well;
- Heal quickly and recover faster;
- Bond with your baby;
- Breastfeed easily, if you choose to do this;

- Be happy and have confidence in your abilities as a mother;
- Get back to pre-pregnancy weight, shape and dimensions very soon after the birth;

The techniques learnt for hypnobirthing are life-long learnings and can be used to improve your life for the better in every aspect – to pass a driving test, to get a new job etc.

Top Ten Tips on How to Create Self-Hypnosis

Thereby tapping into your Inner Power, and using it to be calm, relaxed and in control during your birth

1. **Breathing Method 1**

Breathe in to a count of 4.
Breathe out to a count of 6.
Repeat this as many times as required, and at least fifteen times.

2. **Breathing Method 2**

Breath 1 brings instant mental calmness.
As you breathe out SAY to yourself, "*I am calm*".
Breath 2 brings instant feelings of physical relaxation.
As you breathe out SAY to yourself, "*I am relaxed*".
Breath 3 brings instant feelings of confidence.
As you breathe out SAY to yourself, "*I am confident*"
"*I can do ....*".

By controlling the breath, you automatically lower the adrenalin levels, the panic hormones and release more serotonins, the happy hormone as I call it, which makes you feel good about yourself.

3. **Looking up at the Sky or Ceiling**

This helps release more serotonins which is a morphine based hormone secreted in response to the contractions, relaxing your muscles and body, so taking you to the hypnotic state.

4. **Positive Affirmations**

An affirmation is anything you say or think and this affects your unconscious mind. Your thinking in fact, determines all things. Think negatively and you attract negative realities. Think positively and the benefits you desire in life will come true.

So, say the following affirmations – or change the wording to suit you. An affirmation must be in the present tense and you ask for what you want and not what you don't want.

"I enjoy my pregnancy."

"My digestive system works efficiently and effectively."

"My digestive system is more and more comfortable," (to overcome early morning

sickness).

"I look forward to the birth with excitement."

"I have a wonderfully natural childbirth."

"I heal up easily after the birth."

"I breastfeed easily."

"I enjoy being a mum."

"I trust my instincts and intuition."

Use your imagination and you can make up as many affirmations as you wish.

Emile Coué (1857-1926) put forward the *'Law of Concentrated Attention'*, which states, *"Whenever attention is concentrated on an idea over and over again, it spontaneously tends to realise it."*

5.   Colour that the Unconscious Mind Chooses

This can then be used to visualise the colour flowing over the body from the top of the head right down to the toes, relaxing every muscle, bone, joint, cell, so you are totally relaxed going into the alpha-theta brain pattern of hypnosis and deep relaxation.

6.   Colour can be Used for Healing

The colour, along with positive affirmations, can be used to move the placenta, if it is too low, turn a breech baby, help overcome early morning sickness, boost the immune system and for anything else – even to clear a headache.

7.   Colour to Create a Protective Bubble

By surrounding yourself in your protective bubble of colour, you keep out all negativity from other people, anything you might hear, read or see and also from yourself. This makes you feel, and be, strong, powerful, safe and in control, so you work with your body, and intuition, to give birth easily because you are relaxed and in control.

8.   A Special Place

Allow your unconscious mind to find a place where you feel, and are, truly, deeply comfortable and relaxed. Then go there in your imagination and when you are there, really be there and see what you see, feel what you feel and hear what you hear. When you work with your imagination, your unconscious mind cannot tell the difference between what is real and unreal, so you dissociate from the feelings of the contractions.

You can find your special place and your colour by listening to the free MP3 Relaxation Visualisation, which comes with my App. I've been told that listening to this MP3 at bedtime helps you sleep better too. This will also show you what self-hypnosis is like!
http://hypnosisappstore.com/hypnobirthing/

9.   Visualisation

Visualise the perfect birth, exactly as you want it. When you visualise, then your unconscious mind actualises it. When you visualise, you are using your imagination and this automatically takes you to the daydreaming state of self-hypnosis. Again, you can use this technique for anything – getting the perfect job, house etc.

10.   Listening to a Hypnobirthing CD/MP3

This takes you into hypnosis and installs a programme for birth into your unconscious mind maintaining a calm and relaxed state throughout the pregnancy and birth.

This CD/MP3 is part of the in-App purchase of MP3s and you can find out about my book, which explains the use of the CD/MP3 fully, on the App too.

All these methods are used during pregnancy and for the birth in various combinations, to help you achieve the birth you desire.

If you would like to know more about this topic then please check out my websites:

www.innerpowerhypnobirthing.co.uk
www.birthmadeeasy.co.uk

Why a Caesarean Can be a Positive Birth Experience by Catherine Balavage

I didn't give enough thought to how my son would be born. I just knew it would be painful. I would put the baby clothes we bought, up to my bump and wonder at just how lucky we were to be having a child. It felt like such a happy miracle it didn't even feel real, even as he kicked inside me. Little did I know just how hard his birth would be.

I went into labour with a positive mindset. I am a worrier by nature so I can't say there were not moments when I did not contemplate the worst, but overall, I was feeling strong, happy and positive. We were so excited to finally meet our son. For such a worrier, I wasn't that worried. The human race has survived thousands of years. Women have given birth at home, in caves and even in cars. It was going to hurt but I have always had a high pain threshold. I was confident I could manage the birth. So, when I went into labour on a Sunday evening I did not think it would be long until we met our child. What followed was over eighty hours of hell followed by something glorious: A C-section.

A lot of negativity is said about the C-section. Some people claim it is the easy choice; it isn't, the recovery is a bitch. Others say it isn't natural, it may not be '*natural*' but it has saved countless human lives so hurray for medical science. I, however, have nothing but praise. After eighty hours of labour our son was in distress, the umbilical cord was wrapped around his neck twice and his heartbeat kept on dropping. I switched off and just concentrated on the best-case scenario, knowing that panic would just make the situation worse.

As the surgeon who did my caesarean explained why I should have an emergency caesarean, she looked almost like an angel to me. Within twenty minutes, my son was born. The obstetrician team who did my C-section were amazing (unlike the care I had been given before everything became an emergency). Despite being paralysed from the waist down and being naked underneath my hospital gown, I felt safe. They were truly wonderful and I still think of them when I look at my little boy. My little boy whose life was saved. The midwife even stayed with me the entire time, from the morning when my baby was in distress, until just after noon when he was born. There is an obsession with natural birth these days, and as I was wheeled into the theatre I did feel like I had failed, but the only thing that really matters about childbirth is a healthy mother and child. How that happens doesn't matter in the end, and that is never truer than when they put the baby in your arms. My C-section was not only a positive experience, it saved the life of my son. What could possibly be negative about that?

The Stages of Labour

Labour comes in three stages. Yes, I know, I am sorry. It is a bitch, but you get a baby at the end, so it is worth it. These are the stages:

The first stage is when the contractions open up your cervix at the top of your vagina until you fully dilate to ten centimetres.

The second stage is when you push the baby out.

The third stage is when you deliver the placenta.

These stages are called the latent phase, active labour and the transitional phase.

In the first stages of labour I would stay at home as much as possible. Hospitals are not the best places to have babies. I was even told during my ante-natal class that you should stay at home as much as possible because you might get an infection. It is painful but have some paracetamol and go for a bath or shower. I hate this advice but hot water helps and the paracetamol takes the edge off. Listen to music or try and distract yourself. Learn some breathing techniques either from an ante-natal class, or from a book or CD. The contractions can be hard to get through but you will not be in pain the entire time. Remember that. They come and go in a wave and each one is a step closer to meeting your baby (I also hated it when the midwives told me that! But it has some truth to it. Use it if it helps).

A lot of the advice you get did not work for me, which was to stay active, go for walks, and bounce up and down on a birthing ball. None of this helped make my labour quicker. My advice is rest as much as possible as labour is hard and you need to conserve your energy. If you want to moan, complain, bitch, swear; then do it. Do whatever makes you feel better. I have had many midwives and mothers say it is good to have a glass of wine as labour starts. By all means go for it! Try and do skin to skin contact with your baby as soon as possible. Even if you have a caesarean section. This will help with bonding and breastfeeding.

<u>Some Awesome Tips Unrelated to the Topic of the Book.</u>

The first six weeks with a new-born is brutal, but you will survive it. The first six months is tough as hell, after that things are merely hard. But - and you will not believe me when I say this - try to enjoy it as much as you can. Babies are not babies for long. Very soon they become toddlers, and then you have a whole new set of problems. I look at my son now and I cannot believe how quickly the time went.

Be kind to yourself. Take some time out if you can. Know that you have done something amazing. Making a human being and birthing them is a huge achievement.

Stock up on nappies.

Use all friends and family members who are willing to help. Even if it is just for them to get some shopping.

On the flip side: do not feel selfish if you just want to be alone. It is very intense looking after a child. I think there was a few days after my C-section where I did not even brush my hair, or my teeth. It does not matter if your home is messy, or you are wearing clothes covered in baby sick. Normal service does not have to resume.

It doesn't matter if your child is wearing odd socks.

You will be very tired so sleep as much as you can. Yes, I am going to say it: sleep when your baby sleeps. Or at least try and relax when your baby sleeps. Everything else can wait. You and your health come first.

Do not underestimate how tired you will be. I remember I once made some toast and my son sneezed on it; I was so tired that I just ate it anyway.

If you are breastfeeding then know that it will end and eat as much as you want. It can be difficult to get children to latch at first, but you will get here.

If you are breastfeeding then do not feel guilty. Not all women can. Your child will be fine.

Different Types of Births

You will either give birth in a hospital or at home. You can have a hospital birth in the labour ward, or the midwife led unit usually. If you have had a previous birth with complications you will probably need to give birth in the labour ward. You can have a water birth in a pool at the hospital or at home. Your baby will be born vaginally or by caesarean section. Caesarean sections can be planned or emergency. What kind of birth you can have will change from hospital to hospital. Some do not do planned caesarean sections for example. It is entirely up to you where you want to give birth and how you want to do it. The only person birthing this baby is you. Everyone else is either a spectator or there to offer medical help.

Do not worry about whether you will know whether or not you are in labour. Trust me, it is hard to miss.

Pain Relief Options

The below is my opinion and not medical advice. Talk to your midwife or doctor for any risks associated with medication.

Epidural: Epidurals are as close to God as you can get. They are a bit invasive. You will need a catheter which is not fun, and they require an injection into the spine. But they WORK. They are amazing. One of the best moments of my life was getting an epidural. They do raise the risks of intervention like forceps and caesarean sections, but if you want a pain-free birth it is the only option. Everything else merely takes the edge off.

Pethidine: This is given by injection. It left me dizzy and sick. Make sure that they give you the anti-nausea part too. Otherwise you will just feel very high and very ill. If you can take drugs well I am sure it will be fine. It does leaving you feeling high and can help you sleep.

Gas and Air: Also called Entonox, it is 50% oxygen and 50% nitrous oxide. You breathe this gas in through a mask. Apparently, it takes the edge off but can make you nauseous. The good news is that if you do not like it, it wears off quickly. It is only a mild form of pain relief, and it does not have any effect on the baby. I did not like it and did not think it made a difference. Other mothers swear by it.

TENS machine (Transcutaneous Electric Nerve Stimulation): This is a small machine with pads that stick on your back. It stimulates your nerves with small electric currents. You can turn it up and down. A lot of mums use it for early labour. I have never used one. I have heard both positive and negative things.

Recovering After Birth

Take some time out to recover from the birth. Labour is both physically and emotionally draining. It is very tough indeed. Your tummy will look very squishy and will probably have stretch marks. Do not worry, it will get better. You will bleed for about six weeks after the birth so make sure you buy some maternity pads. This will happen whether you have a caesarean section or a normal birth. You will have some afterpains and it might hurt to sit down. Especially if you have had stitches. If you had a caesarean section you will need to wear compression stockings and inject medication for seven days so you do not get blood clots. You will have a catheter for twenty-four hours. If you need to cough then hold a pillow to your scar, it helps with the pain. Your stitches will probably dissolve but might be the type that need to be removed. Take paracetamol if you are in pain. When in the hospital, do not be scared to say if you are not coping with the pain or you need anything. You will need lots of help with lifting and moving. Get as much help as possible. Get other people to lift your baby up and hand them to you. You will not be able to drive for a few weeks. Buy some big knickers that will go over your scar line. And do not worry about your scar, it will fade in time.

It is normal to feel a bit sad or over emotional after the first few days of having a baby. Do not worry about it, but if your mood does not lift then go to the health visitor or your GP. There is a lot of help out there. You are never alone.

What You Will Need

For you: your birth notes, warm comfortable clothes, a dressing gown will be handy, pyjamas, a top you can easily breastfeed in, a breastfeeding cover, slippers, a breastfeeding bra and breast pads, maternity pads and spare underwear, a towel and toiletries, drinks and snacks to keep up your energy, money for parking if you drive, an iPod or iPad, a camera and some books or magazines.

For baby: Moses basket, cot, nappies, blanket, grow-bag, baby grows, sleep suits, hats, socks and booties, scratch mits, a baby bath, muslin squares, baby wipes, baby change mat, anti-bacterial gel and nappy bags. You may also want a cuddly toy. Make sure it is suitable from birth. Also, be careful with the nappy bags as they can suffocate children.

You will need either a sling or a pram to carry baby around in. Maybe both. If you have had a caesarean section you will not be able to carry the baby around in a sling. You will also need a car seat if you use a car at any point. You can take the pram in a black cab.

You have forty-two days to register your baby's birth in England, Northern Ireland and Wales, and twenty-one days in Scotland. Make sure you do not forget!

Good luck with your labour, and with your new life as a parent. I wish you all the best, and I hope this book was helpful in some way. Always remember: you are a warrior. You have created life and you are amazing. Keep in touch with me on Twitter at @Balavage. I would love to know how you are getting on. There is so much help and wonderful people out there. Join baby classes, join toddler groups and go to the park. Download an app like Mush and get in touch with other mothers. Being a mother is a privilege but it is hard. Do not worry though, we are all here for you.

Other books by the same author

How To Be a Successful Actor: Becoming an Actorpreneur
The Wedding Survival Guide: How To Plan Your Big Day Without Losing Your Sanity
The Ultimate Guide To Becoming a Successful Blogger
What Do You Think? A Collection of Poems

About The Author

Catherine Balavage is an author, writer, editor and actor. She is the founder and editor of Frost Magazine. She has written two novels which she is currently editing, and four non-fiction books. Catherine lives in South-West London with her husband James and their children.

If you enjoyed this book then please leave a review for it on Amazon or Goodreads. Thank you.

www.ingramcontent.com/pod-product-compliance
Lightning Source LLC
Chambersburg PA
CBHW060804260726
48660CB00002B/767